SELLING HEALING

The intersections between arts, creativity and health are of significant importance in the humanities and social sciences. Arts and health research, for example, suggests that the arts offer participatory and transformational alternatives to traditional health communication. However, concepts and methods are predominantly informed by Global North research, and critical insights from arts traditions elsewhere remain to be fully integrated into common models. Ghana offers a unique case study for examining local and global dynamics in arts-based health communication, because of the country's rich art traditions as well as its place in global history and in the global imagination. Healing art forms like music and sculpture have evolved through intentional cross-cultural borrowings, as well as through changes imposed through slavery, colonialism and post-colonial political systems. *Selling Healing* tells a polyvocal story of how Ghanaian art forms intersect with health, illness and healing, inviting a re-imagining of health communication in global health.

AMA DE-GRAFT AIKINS is Professor of Social Psychology at the University of Ghana and a Visiting Professor at the London School of Economics. She was a British Academy Global Professor, based at University College London's Institute of Advanced Studies, between 2019 and 2023.

SELLING HEALING

Creative Arts and Health Communication in Ghana

AMA DE-GRAFT AIKINS

University College London

CAMBRIDGE
UNIVERSITY PRESS

CAMBRIDGE
UNIVERSITY PRESS

Shaftesbury Road, Cambridge CB2 8EA, United Kingdom

One Liberty Plaza, 20th Floor, New York, NY 10006, USA

477 Williamstown Road, Port Melbourne, VIC 3207, Australia

314–321, 3rd Floor, Plot 3, Splendor Forum, Jasola District Centre, New Delhi – 110025, India

103 Penang Road, #05-06/07, Visioncrest Commercial, Singapore 238467

Cambridge University Press is part of Cambridge University Press & Assessment, a department of the University of Cambridge.

We share the University's mission to contribute to society through the pursuit of education, learning and research at the highest international levels of excellence.

www.cambridge.org
Information on this title: www.cambridge.org/9781009244435

DOI: 10.1017/9781009244459

When citing this work, please include a reference to the DOI 10.1017/9781009244459

First published 2025

A catalogue record for this publication is available from the British Library

A Cataloging-in-Publication data record for this book is available from the Library of Congress

ISBN 978-1-009-24443-5 Hardback

To the memory of my beloved parents, Seth and Eleanor de-Graft Aikins.

Contents

List of Figures, Tables and Boxes — *page* viii
Acknowledgements — x
Abbreviations — xii

1 Introduction — 1
2 If You Sell Your Sickness You Get a Cure — 22
3 Mr Wise and Mr Foolish Go to Town — 47
4 All Die (No) Be Die — 58
5 Food Is Medicine, Food Is Poison — 77
6 Out of Your Mind — 96
7 We Cannot Eat Stories — 115
8 Colonial Virus — 131
9 Conclusions — 153

Appendix 1: Map Showing Sites of Arts-Based Interventions — 163
Appendix 2: Interviews — 166
Appendix 3: Selected Primary and Secondary Data — 168
References — 188
Index — 202

Figures, Tables and Boxes

Figures

Frontispiece Wood sculpture of the Sankofa bird

1.1 An Akan Drum *page* 5

2.1 Pluralistic healthcare facilities in Ga Mashie in 2014 31

2.2 'Pampi' at the entry gate of the Ga Mashie Chief Priest's Compound 34

2.3 Mural on the wall of the Ga Mashie Chief Priest's Compound 35

2.4 Ga Mashie Chief Priest and his team 35

2.5 Diabetes Last Stop signpost, Tema 38

2.6 Shiloh Herbal wall advert, Kintampo 39

2.7 Agbeve Tonic van, Osu, Accra 41

2.8 Agbeve Tonics approved by the FDA 41

3.1 'No bathing allowed without suits' cartoon, *Gold Coast Leader* 51

4.1 AIDS Is Real billboard 62

4.2 'Do you want to be like this' AIDS signpost 63

5.1 RHN signpost outside Hohoe District Hospital 82

5.2 A bowl of fufu and palm nut soup 87

5.3 Women selling ultra processed foods in front of an RHN signpost, Amasaman Health Centre 88

5.4 Pepsi Homowo poster, Ga Mashie, Accra 91

5.5 KFC billboard, George Walker Bush Highway, Accra 92

5.6 Indomie Billboard, George Walker Bush Highway, Accra 93

6.1 Schematic layout of the Out of Your Mind exhibition 99

6.2 Spaced Out, painting by Wiz Kudowor 100

6.3 Metaphoric Boundaries, painting by Amenyo Dzikunu-Bansah 101

6.4 Vagrant writings on a wall, Takoradi, photograph by Rikki Wemega-Kwawu 103

6.5 'A view of Danso's junk treasure trove', Tema, photograph by Bernard Akoi-Jackson 103

6.6 Woman in a prayer camp, Kintampo, photograph by Ursula Read 105
6.7 Casting out evil spirits in a Pentecostal church, Kintampo, photograph by Ursula Read 105
6.8 Man with a log, Kintampo, photograph by Ursula Read 106
6.9 Shoeshine Boy, painting by Kwame 107
6.10 Woman in Dress, painting by Yaganoma Baatoulkuu and a group of patients 108
6.11 For Larson, painting by Bernard Akoi-Jackson 110
7.1 Nana Yaa Agyeman with ShareCare Ghana (SCG) members 121
7.2 Christopher Agbeba with children from SCG and Jamestown Children's Health Club 124
7.3 Marching for World Hypertension Day 127
8.1 Chaotic COVID-19, painting by Agyei Agyemang 132
8.2 Coronavirus Greetings, cartoon by Tilapia da Cartoonist 134
8.3 'Apio Sanitizer', cartoon by Akosua 134
8.4 COVID-19 mural, painted by Ghana Graffiti Collective 140
8.5 'Chale Covid Still De', COVID-19 mural painted by Hamid Nii Nortey 140
8.6 Bernard Akoi-Jackson in a face mask made by Jenesus Clothing 141
8.7 'Lockdown', featuring the aeroplane motif, GTP COVID-19 textile design 145
8.8 'Fellow Ghanaians', featuring the eye glasses motif, GTP COVID-19 textile design 145
8.9 'No more free food after lockdown', cartoon by Tilapia da Cartoonist 147
8.10 'Balanced diet versus balanced pockets', cartoon by Makaveli 147
8.11 'Dumsor-COVID-19 economy comparison', cartoon by Tilapia da Cartoonist 148
9.1 Arts and health communication ecosystem in Ghana 158

Tables

7.1 Patient support groups for chronic diseases in Ghana 126

Boxes

2.1 'How Ghana Herbal Hospitals Advertise Themselves on TV'. Excerpt of a comedy sketch 44

Acknowledgements

The idea for this book evolved from a paper I wrote on COVID-19 arts in Ghana, that was published in 2020 by the *Journal of the British Academy*. I have to start by thanking Philip Lewis, Head of International at the British Academy, who encouraged me to write the paper, and Stephen Acerra, Psychology and Neuroscience editor at Cambridge University Press, who found its abstract on a conference website and suggested there might be more to write on arts and health in Ghana.

As I fleshed out the book proposal, a deeper reserve of ideas emerged from years of engaging with artists, art patrons and art educators in Ghana. I remembered conversations and collaborations with, especially, Frances Ademola, Bernard Akoi-Jackson, Panji Anoff, Fatric Bewong, Grace Brew-Appiah, Kwamina Ewusie, Ablade Glover, Wiz Kudowor, Kofi Setordji, Collins Seymah Smith, Odile Tevie and Kati Torda. I had always wanted to showcase these 'off-duty' relationships in my 'day job' of psychological and health research: suddenly I found a way.

I wrote the book during my time as a British Academy Global Professor at University College London (UCL)'s Institute of Advanced Studies (IAS). My research project for the Global Professorship, which generated writing material, was generously funded by the British Academy. IAS gave me an intellectual home to think, develop the project, and write. I thank my IAS mentor Megan Vaughan, two directors Tamar Garb and Nicola Miller, and Catherine Stokes, IAS's administrator and my go-to guru on all things UCL.

I was supported by an ad hoc, but superb, team – Jemima Okai, Vida Asah-Ayeh, Francis Agyei, Paapa Yaw Asante, Ernestina Tetteh – who helped me to conduct new interviews, translate and transcribe text, gather archival material, and commission, acquire and photograph art objects.

Trisha Greenhalgh involved me in a series of writing and speaking projects, which led to two years of teaching a class on 'arts and health communication in African contexts' on her Oxford MSc Course in

Translational Science and Global Health and on Martin Bauer's MSc Course in Health Communication at my alma mater, the London School of Economics and Political Science. Three anonymous reviewers reviewed my proposal and the final manuscript and provided critical and insightful comments, at each stage. These academic relationships, old and new, helped to sharpen my ideas and place the Ghanaian material in global context.

Thank you to friends and family who heard variations of chapters I was working on, who debated ideas with me, and who supported the writing process without even knowing they were by filling the void my mother left in November 2022: Baba and Shirley Abu, Charles Agyemang, Daniel Kojo Arhinful, Kobina and Ama Anin, Adote Anum, Yaw Awuku Boohene, Delroy Corinaldi, Flora Cornish, Kwadwo and Naa Koram, Naa Adaawah and Bob Kumi, Akua and Hoffman Lartey, Hélène Neveu Kringelbach, Kathryn Nwajiaku-Dahou, Misan and Ije Nwokorie, Louise Owusu-Kwarteng and, to constant anchors, my great-aunt Doris Anin and uncle Barfuor Adjei-Barwuah.

To Yaa and Nana Amankwah and Terrence Hibbert, I did quite a bit of writing, reading, thinking, talking and de-stressing in your homes: I cannot thank you enough for the sanctuary.

Abbreviations

AHDA	- African Hebrew Development Agency
AHIC	- African Hebrew Israelite Community
AMA	- Accra Metropolitan Assembly
BBC	- British Broadcasting Corporation
CBT	- cognitive behavioural therapy
CCG	- Christian Council of Ghana
CHPS	- community-based health planning and services
COVAX	- COVID-19 Vaccines Global Access
CPMR	- Centre for Plant Medicine Research
DANIDA	- Danish International Development Agency
DFID	- Department for International Development
EU	- European Union
FAO	- Food and Agriculture Organization
FDA	- Food and Drugs Authority
FHI	- Family Health International
GAAS	- Ghana Academy of Arts and Sciences
GAC	- Ghana AIDS Commission
GBC	- Ghana Broadcasting Corporation
GFD	- Ghana Federation of Disability Organisations
GGC	- Ghana Graffiti Collective
GhNCDA	- Ghana Non-communicable Disease Alliance
GHS	- Ghana Health Service
GNCFC	- Ghana National Canoe Fisherman Council
GoG	- Government of Ghana
GSA	- Ghana Standards Authority
GTA	- Ghana Tourism Authority
GTP	- Ghana Textiles Printing
GTV	- Ghana Television
IMF	- International Monetary Fund
IOM	- International Organization for Migration

JHU	- Johns Hopkins University
KNUST	- Kwame Nkrumah University of Science and Technology
LSHTM	- London School of Hygiene and Tropical Medicine
MDGs	- Millennium Development Goals
MEHSOG	- Mental Health Society of Ghana
MIFAD	- Ministry of Fisheries and Aquaculture Development
MOFA	- Ministry of Food and Agriculture
MOGCSP	- Ministry of Gender, Children and Social Protection
MOH	- Ministry of Health
NCD Alliance	- Non-communicable Disease Alliance
NCDCP	- Non-communicable Disease Control Programme
NDC	- National Democratic Congress
NFPTA	- National Fish Processors & Traders Association
NMIMR	- Noguchi Memorial Institute for Medical Research
NPP	- National Patriotic Party
PAR	- participatory action research
PLWHA	- people living with HIV/AIDS
PLWNCDS	- people living with noncommunicable diseases
PPAG	- Planned Parenthood of Ghana
SDGs	- Sustainable Development Goals
TAMD	- Traditional and Alternative Medicine Directorate
UCC	- University of Cape Coast
UG	- University of Ghana
UNICEF	- United Nations Children's Fund
USAID	- United States Agency for International Development
UTV	- United Television
WACCBIP	- West African Centre for Cell Biology of Infectious Pathogens
WB	- World Bank
WHO	- World Health Organization

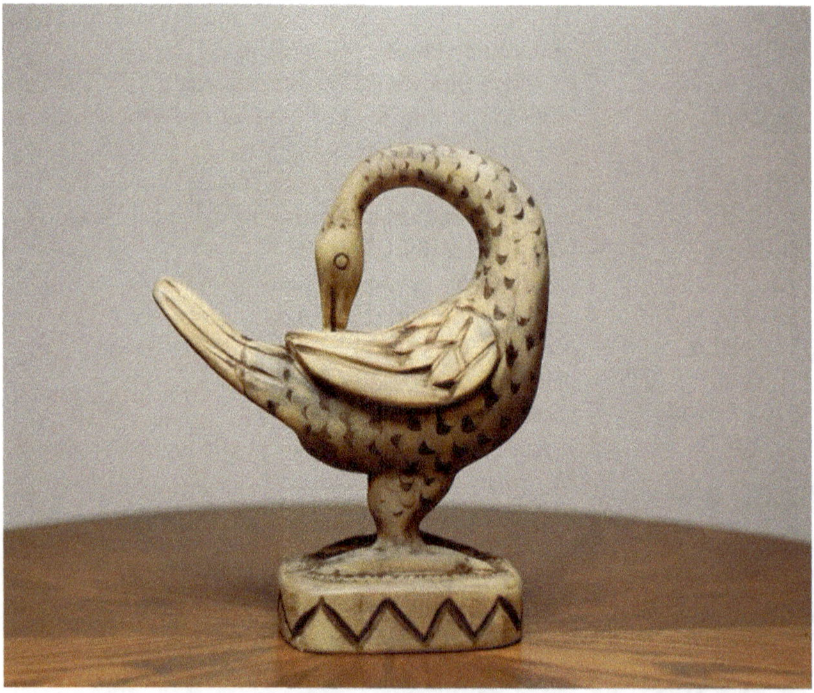

Sankofa bird. Commissioned reproduction of an old Akan wood sculptural design, carved from Tweneboa wood by Hamza Ibrahim, August 2023.

CHAPTER 1

Introduction

The gods may be considered patrons of the arts.

Irene Odotei (2016)

Creative arts drive Ghanaian social life. Singing, drumming, dancing, drama, body art, sculpture, painting, textile design and other art forms are woven into significant life events such as the celebration of births, the marking of puberty, the formalisation of marriage and the mourning of death.

In many Ghanaian communities, the arts also inform everyday practices in ways that generate well-being and health at individual and social levels.

In Fante communities along the southern coast, women who supported warrior Asafo companies – military groups that led battles against European slavers and colonists – belonged to singing groups called *adzewa*.[1] Initially formed to exhort male warriors and to fight alongside them when the situation demanded, they now perform for themselves and their broader communities, telling stories about community and women's health through satire, song and dance.[2]

In Sirigu, in the Upper East Region, women have painted on walls for centuries, in a tradition called "bambolse", meaning "embellished, decorated, or made more attractive" in the Nankam language.[3] These muralists use clay, tree barks, rocks and other natural materials sourced in their local environment. They draw in geometric shapes that trace the contours of bodies and everyday objects and paint only with the colours red, brown, black and white, creating public art that beautifies their households and

[1] Esi Sutherland-Addy (1998) notes that in the Oguaa-Edina (Cape Coast-Elmina) area, *adzewa* is a major lyrical form "dominated by women as composers and performers" (p.1).

[2] Kingsley Ampomah (2014, p.119) discusses a song by a Winneba group, titled *Awomawu*. The song tells the story of a woman called Efua, who experiences repeated baby loss, and it pays tribute to "women who live with the painful experience of losing their children soon after birth".

[3] Sela Adjei (2020) quoting Perani and Smith (1998, p.7). See also Rhoda Woets (2014).

communities.[4] As they paint their walls, they sing and dance, drawing comfort and strength from their social bonds in similar ways to the Fante adzewa groups.[5]

Every ethnic group in Ghana commemorates its origin story and notable achievements through annual festivals. Festivals run over several days – following weeks of preparation – and bring people of all ages and social statuses together into the public domain: children, youth, adults, the elderly, chiefs, priests, local political figures and in some cases community outcasts such as individuals living with mental illness or physical disabilities.

American art historians Herbert M. Cole and Doran H. Ross (1977) describe these festivals as 'art events'.

> [T]ime, people and scale are the components which lift individual objects and festival activities into the realm of art. [...] Multitudes of objects, decorated people, dances, skits and sacrifices transform a once quiet space into an arena of [colour], sound and motion. The festival embraces the community, raising both people and place onto a plane marked by aesthetic, spiritual and social values (p.200).

They observe, rightly, that it is during festivals that indigenous art forms come to life. Static objects with circumscribed functions for specified groups of people such as chiefs, healers, youth and new mothers shift to "kinetic sculpture" (p.200), taking on new, dynamic meanings and functions for all present:

> [A]rt [...] becomes kinetic sculpture during a festival. Asafo flags are thrown and swirled in dance; pottery, stools, and chairs are carried in processions, architecture becomes a backdrop in shrine rituals and sometimes as sculpture to climb on. Drums tell of history, sing praises, and beat out proverbs. Jewellery and dress shift constantly – flowing in dance, blending with other patterns of personal decoration or setting them off. This activation of Ghanaian art is an important form of its quality (p.200).

Festivals are also spaces for subverting social and cultural norms for personal and community health and well-being. Individuals and social groups can speak truth to power without fear of punishment and seek

[4] The late Ghanaian artist and art historian Atta Kwami was inspired by indigenous Ghanaian art forms. In a tribute his widow Pamela Clarkson-Kwami wrote for him in the *UK Guardian*, she recalls he studied "the northern murals that the women paint – that is amazing. There was one woman and she painted abstract shapes. Atta asked her where she got them, and she said 'I sit on the roof and look at the cows'" (Guardian, 5 September 2022).

[5] Personal communication, Fatric Bewong, December 2021.

redress for past psychosocial harms. "When a man has spoken freely thus", notes Peter Kwasi Sarpong (1967) citing R. S. Rattray (1955), "he will feel his *sunsum* ('personality, character, energy') cool and quieted, and the *sunsum* of the other person against whom he has now openly spoken will be quieted also".

Activating Art in Healing

The 'aesthetic, spiritual and social values' displayed in festivals are embodied in indigenous healing systems. These systems also "activate art" to serve their professional purposes. Traditional shrine architecture and artefacts are designed to prepare clients psychologically for the healing process. Wall reliefs in Asante and Tallensi shrines, for instance, depict animals associated with health and protection in local folklore.[6] Mural art on Ewe shrines depicts symbols of healing through abstract motifs painted with mixed materials, some ordinary (paint), some symbolic (mud, blood, alcohol).[7] Diagnostic and healing objects in various ethnic traditions such as amulets and wooden figurines are imbued with the dynamic energy of small gods.

Diagnosis by an Asante shrine priest, Dagomba diviner or Ewe priestess might be accompanied by performance: a song, dance or drumming by master drummers using specific sets of communicative ('talking') drums – the Asante *atumpan* or Dagomba *lungi*. The healer might wear art on their body, such as intricate patterns drawn or stamped into skin with white clay, or a specially designed attire stitched with ritually significant artefacts such as beads, cowrie shells or feathers. The treatment processes may likely involve a similar deployment of bodily art on the client or guided ritual performance.

Specially trained artists are commissioned to produce indigenous healing arts. Fante Posuban shrines are built only by artists who have been trained to understand the customs of the target Fante community as well

[6] British psychologist turned anthropologist Meyer Fortes, who conducted research in Tallensi (or Frafra) communities in the 1930s, dismissed the wall art of female muralists but noted the artistic merit of Tallensi shrine art: "The women sometimes decorated the walls of a room with lozenge-like blobs and irregular lines of chevrons, but the nearest thing to a work of art would have been the spread-eagle flat bas-relief of a crocodile or chameleon very crudely modelled in mud on the surface of some ancestor shrines" (Fortes, 1981, p.47). Akan clans have animals as symbols of identity and protection – each chosen for specific qualities. For instance, among the Fante, the Aduana clan has a dog, which symbolises honesty and industriousness; the Asona clan has the crow, which symbolises statesmanship and patriotism.

[7] Adjei (2020).

as the importance of ecological balance in their spiritual lives (Labi, 2019). Asante woodcarvers know what kinds of wood to select for stools (ɔsɛsɛ) or drums (*tweneboa*), due to the 'intrinsic supernatural character' of each wood, and how to propitiate the gods before felling trees (Sarpong, 1967). The women who paint murals on Ewe shrine walls master abstract painting techniques of "dripping, soak-staining, smudging, sprinkling, stencilling, dabbing, splattering and splashing" as well as an understanding of the spiritual dimensions of the materials – "mud, blood, alcohol" – they use (Adjei, 2020, p.172).

A central feature of arts traditions is that they are driven by strategic cultural borrowing. Dagomba drums beat Akan proverbs (Kinney, 1970). Akan art forms – for example, gold weights, stools, textiles and ceramic pots – incorporate elements "actively borrowed" through cross-cultural encounters, including with itinerant Muslim traders from West African countries (Cole and Ross, 1977, p.214). Strategic cultural borrowing is also a core feature in indigenous healing arts. Ghanaian historian Irene Odotei (2016) provides a clear example in her juxtaposition of arts in Ga social life and arts in Ga healing traditions:

> [T]he Ga people give us a good example of borrowing and utilising materials from other sources. If you go to the annual Homowo festival of the La people, they have the category of the *Kpa* songs, which have their characteristic rhythms played by drums supposed to be deities and played only once a year. [They] are supposed to be vessels which narrate the history and expound the philosophy of the people. The proverbs used to embellish a song are usually borrowed from Akan, Ewe, or even English. When you look at our traditional religion too, [...] you will find *nme*, *kplee*, *akon*, *otu* and *tigare*.[8] [The deities] will show you the origin of the people who composed a song. They are all now Ga. When the singers are not possessed, they cannot speak the special language of mediums. It is only when they are under possession that you will discover this creativity. I think that the gods may be considered patrons of the arts, in this sense that they are making sure that human beings express what is in them and sing to that effect (p.165).

Masters of Re-Inventing (Healing) Traditions

Indigenous healing systems and the arts they activate are as old as the oldest Ghanaian community. These systems existed before coastal communities engaged with European imperial trade in the late fifteenth century. During the brutal and dehumanising era of the transatlantic slave

[8] *nme*, *kplee*, *akon*, *otu* and *tigare* are deities.

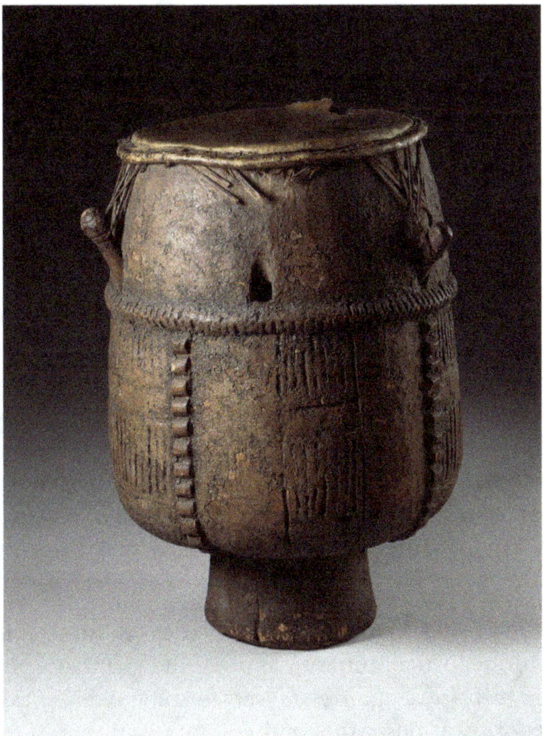

Figure 1.1 An Akan drum displayed at the British Museum (©The Trustees of the British Museum).

trade, spanning the late fifteenth century until the early nineteenth century, indigenous arts tempered chronic suffering and strengthened social bonds. Psychotherapeutic art forms like drumming, singing and trance-induced dancing helped enslaved men, women and children cope during the journey from the hinterland to the coast and through the Middle Passage (see Figure 1.1).[9]

[9] For the British Museum's series titled *Objects of Crisis*, African-American writer Bonnie Greer recounted how one 'Akan Drum' entered the museum's collection (see Figure 1.1). "The Akan drum was found in what is now Virginia, and it was found in [...] the mid-18th century, and up until maybe 70/80 years ago, it was thought to be an indigenous object because the skin is deer skin, which is from Virginia, and so it was [...] put in the Americas section of the British Museum. And then [...] the British Museum [...] started to look, test, and realized that the wood and the cork, which holds up the skin across the drum is actually from West Africa, so it can't be an indigenous American object. It is actually a West African object, which was amazing to discover and then the next thing they pieced together [...] was how did it get to Virginia? Well, the only explanation for it getting

Art forms used in battles and wars, such as messages communicated through drums, horns, song and dance, were also used as communication tools during the many revolts that were executed by the enslaved on slave ships during the Middle Passage. These arts traditions were transported to the New World and formed the basis of healing traditions in the Caribbean and among African-American communities in the American South.[10]

Initially, indigenous healing systems co-existed peacefully with the medical systems of imperial traders and, further down the line, with colonial medicine. American anthropologist Adam Mohr (2009) describes an example of a "therapeutically inclusive model" between the Akan indigenous healing system (what he terms 'Akan therapeutics') and colonial medicine in nineteenth-century Akwapim towns –present-day Eastern Region – where the first Basel missionaries from Germany settled and converted Akan communities to Christianity. The prevalent conditions in these towns were smallpox, measles, whooping cough, malaria, skin infections, leprosy and dysentery. Akan therapeutics was a highly structured system with four categories of specialists, whose practices often intersected:

(1) Priests (*asofo*, sing. *osofo*) served old deities (abosom, sing. *obosom*) and performed ritual duties to appease the guardian spirit;
(2) Prophets (*akomfo*, sing. *okomfo*) served some old deities and were conduits of spirit possession and communication;
(3) Medicine makers (*aduruyefo*, sing. *oduruyefo*) specialised in making medicines (*aduru*) to treat a broad range of 'personal afflictions and social situations';
(4) Herbalists (*adunsifo*, sing. *odunsifo*) made medicine from roots and herbs, focusing on pharmacological properties, although the spiritual element could also be used.

Healing involved diagnosing and treating the underlying spiritual dimensions of disease and social crises. This system was more effective than

to Virginia and being in the collection of Hans Sloan eventually was that it must have crossed over on a slave ship with my ancestors" (visit: (664) *Objects of Crisis: The Akan drum* – YouTube).

At the British Museum, the drum (see Figure 1.1) is displayed in the North America section and belongs to museum objects placed under the category of "Collecting and Empire".

[10] Margarite Fernandez Olmos and Lizabeth Paravisini-Gebert (2022) document the influence of West African healing traditions, via enslaved communities of Ewe, Fon and Yoruba heritage, on Haitian Vodou religion. See also Freddi Williams Evans (2011) on the West African provenance of drums played in Congo Square in New Orleans; and Sharon F. Patton (1998) on the influence of "African culture: ceremonies, house plans and folk art" (p.285) on plantation life in the American South.

biomedicine for the local population as well as for the European missionaries. Mohr tells the story of two Basel missionaries – Andreas Riis and Johannes Zimmerman[11] – who were cured of their illnesses through Akan therapeutics after treatment by biomedical doctors failed. One of them, Andreas Riis, claimed that "Dr. Tietz, the European physician in Christianborg, was useless [because] all patients [he] treated died, while those treated by the local healer survived" (p.445).

In other locations across the country, a subset of medicine makers and herbalists, such as bonesetters and midwives, provided superior treatment that rivalled biomedical systems.

However, as colonial medicine absorbed the systemic race-based shift in Western sciences – the era of scientific racism – collaboration turned to violent domination.[12] Throughout the colonial era, from 1874 to 1957 (in the Gold Coast), there were sustained attempts to devalue and destroy indigenous healing knowledge systems and practices, even as new medical methods and materials drew on these very systems. Successive colonial administrations banned drumming, singing, dancing and other arts-based traditions underpinning healing rituals and practices, as well as social customs such as puberty rites.[13] 'Colonial subjects' who defied the bans faced hefty fines and, in extreme cases, imprisonment, exile and state-sanctioned killings.[14] The same methods of violent domination and erasure, it is worth noting, were deployed over the same period by plantation owners and colonial authorities in the Caribbean and the American South.[15]

[11] Johannes Zimmerman 'wrote the first Ga dictionary and translated the first Ga Bible' (Mohr, 2009, p.445).

[12] In *'Race', Racism and Psychology*, British historian of psychology Graham Richards (1997) observes that by the time psychology was "cohering as a discipline" in the late nineteenth century, much was "apparently 'known' about African inferiority" (p.16). Richards identifies four distinct attitudes and approaches displayed by key theorists towards Africa and Africans at the time: the 'benignly paternal, the blithely imperial, the elaborately scientistic and the semi-mystical and protofascist'. These attitudes extended beyond African targets, to non-Western cultures more generally and informed theories and methods in imperial science, medicine, psychiatry and associated disciplines on race differences and human development, that are now labelled as 'Scientific Racism'.

[13] See Akyeampong (1995), Mohr (2009), Parker (2000).

[14] Possibly the most violent display of colonial power was when the Asantehene Prempeh I and his family were exiled to the Seychelles in 1896 – two years after the bloody Anglo-Asante 'Sagrenti' war that claimed 4,000 Asante lives – and the Asante Odwira festival was banned until their return decades later in 1924 (Parker, 2000, p.217).

[15] When enslaved communities in Trinidad and Tobago were prevented from playing skin drums by British colonial administrators and plantation owners in the 1880s, they improvised with materials in their environment and created drums made from bamboo, called 'tamboo bamboo'. Decades later, in the 1930s, experimentations with biscuit tins, dustbins, paint tins and old metal containers

Anthropologists observe that African indigenous healers are masters of re-inventing tradition. The core motivation to re-invent, it is argued, is a response to the critical demands of communities with health needs. British anthropologist Murray Last (1981) notes, in his ethnographic study of Hausa medicine in Northern Nigeria in the 1960s, that where healing was concerned, people voted with their feet, and healers who did not deliver solutions became irrelevant and eventually went out of business. Similar observations have been made of the precarious lifespans of shrines in colonial Gold Coast (Field, 1937; Goody, 1987). Among the Dagara in Ghana's Upper West Region, the weaknesses of existing healing systems drove "the search for new shrines, new curing agencies" (Goody, 1987, p.156). Across several ethnic groups, there is a cultural imperative to 'sell one's sickness in order to get a cure': "*wo ton wo yareɛ a na wonya n'ano aduro*" (Twi). When illness strikes, this imperative drives healer-shopping: the use of multiple healers without referral from previous healers for a single episode of illness (Kroeger, 1983). Healer-shopping is in turn shaped by assessment of the best options available in the pluralistic health marketplace: clients assess healers' technical knowledge of health conditions, their diagnostic and treatment expertise, and how accessible they are geographically as well as culturally and financially. Healing environments are therefore co-constructed by healers and their clients, and these environments are dynamic because they respond to societal health needs, which are in turn shaped by wider epidemiological and socio-economic trends.

But it is important to note that the motivation to re-invent healing traditions is not only driven by internal sociopsychological factors. It is also shaped by external socio-political forces. Before and during the colonial era, communities and chiefs rebelled against the excesses of British governance, using strategies of non-compliance, defiance and physical battle (Addo-Fening, 2013).[16] In the same way, indigenous healers had to change and innovate with an eye to material and existential threats from

led to the invention of the steelpan – the percussion instrument at the heart of calypso and soca music (Personal communication, Jeff Klein, March 2023; see Kim Johnson (2011) for a detailed history). Similarly, the contemporary American drum set traces its lineage to early drum sets made from cans and other found materials by enslaved communities in the American South who were banned from playing their traditional skin drums (Cataliotti, 2022).

[16] In *The Makings of a Diplomatist*, the former diplomat Alexander Quaison-Sackey recounts a story of rebellion in Winneba (his hometown) in 1812 against the British Commander of the Winneba fort, James Meredith (Quaison-Sackey, 2021). Meredith had dispatched community 'gold and other valuables' to England and refused to return them despite several appeals by chiefs and elders. One Sunday morning, "the Commander was seized and taken to the prickly grasslands, where he was made to walk barefoot while the people beat drums and chanted war songs. Meredith died as a result of this harsh treatment" (p.5). The British government – through a 'Man of War' sent from

adversarial and increasingly violent colonial European administrative policies. And because they were under constant threat, they had to be creative, and their creativity had to be subversive. Indigenous healing systems have survived and thrived in large part, particularly over the last century, due to these creative strategies.

Selling Healing

In *Selling Healing*, I aim to tell a polyvocal story of how the arts intersect with health, illness and healing in Ghana at multiple levels of social organisation, from the local to the geopolitical. The story will have three intersecting strands.

The first strand will build on my opening argument – that arts drive Ghanaian social life – by demonstrating that arts are a core feature of health communication in Ghanaian communities. Following social psychologists Catherine Campbell and Kerry Scott (2011, p.267), I define health communication as "*any form of communication* that seeks to empower people to take control over their health". I include arts as a fundamental form of communication in healing environments.

Daisy Fancourt and Saoirse Finn (2019, p.1) offer a succinct definition of art, from the arts and health field:

> [T]he art object (whether physical or experiential) [is] valued in its own right rather than merely as a utility; provid[es] imaginative experiences for both the producer and audience; and compris[es] or provoke[es] an emotional response. In addition, the production of art is characterized by requiring novelty, creativity or originality; requiring specialized skills; and relating to the rules of form, composition or expression.

While this definition draws on cross-cultural references, the sources are predominantly Euro-American. In the interdisciplinary field of African art history, art, as defined by indigenous African (arts) communities, has some features that are aligned with the Euro-American characterisation, and others that diverge. The production of art in African contexts is also "characterized by requiring novelty, creativity or originality and specialized skills relating to the rules of form, composition or expression". But

Freetown, Sierra Leone – retaliated by destroying the fort and only spared the townsfolk after a peace offering of gold. Today, Winneba has a Meredith Street, and a Methodist Church stands in place of the fort. "Once every year the people drum the same message [they sent] to James Meredith on that fateful Saturday in 1812: 'tomorrow we shall kill James' (*Okyena Kwesi, yebokum* James) repeated many times during the annual Deer Hunt (*Aboakyer*) Festival" (pp.5–6).

depending on the kind of art being produced, other forces are at play. To produce sacred art objects, for example, specialised skills are required, as we saw for Asante woodcarvers and Fante Posuban shrine artists. But these art forms truly come to life when spirits and forces of the invisible world move the artist. As Odotei (2016, p.165) observed of Ga ritual singers, "when the singers are not possessed, they cannot speak the special language of mediums. It is only when they are under possession that you will discover this creativity". Similarly, the Malian historian Amadou Hampate Ba (1976, p.16) observes of the Nyamakala, a class of Bambara craftsmen that include woodworkers (who make ritual objects including masks) and griots (public entertainers who compose music, sing, dance and tell stories): "the craftsman needed to be in a state of mind which matched the moment of its creation. Sometimes, he would go into a trance, and when he emerged from it, he would create". The difference between the secular and sacred art object, Ba (1976, p.16) notes, is that the "secular object is not 'consecrated' and therefore not 'loaded' with spiritual energy".

Secondly, theorists observe that the distinctions created between art and craft in European contexts do not exist in African contexts: "the unpredictable, culture-transcending element of creativity in artistic production" operates on the same plane as craftwork which is "predictable, traditional, competent but limited by precept and technique" (Polakoff, 1978, p.22). Therefore, the art object, whether physical or experiential, can be valued in its own aesthetic right (art for art's sake, arts as essential for survival) as well as a utility (art for everyday use).

Thirdly, the production of art is participatory. In the realms of healing, for example, American art historian Suzanne Preston Blier (1993) observes "the complex interweave of individuals who both participate in the creative process as artists – diviners, ritual activators and the like – and bring signification to the work through their divergent roles as viewers, users, worshippers and caretakers" (p.147). The art object therefore provides imaginative experiences for both the producer and a participating audience. And across several communities, participating audiences express a preference for multi-form arts: for example, "visual arts [. . .] music, dance and oral performance" (Ben-Amos, 1989, p.39) in combination, rather than in isolation.

Finally, art is "grounded in social life [. . .] fully entrenched in the variant and varying societal roots which make and frame it" (Blier, 1993, p.154). Art therefore communicates at the various registers of social life – such as political, economic, educational, recreational and religious (Ba,

1976; Barber, 1987). Because social life operates on cognitive, emotional, physical, social and spiritual levels, art comprises and provokes these multilayered responses. In moments of deep connection between artists and their participating audience, these multilayered responses may transform the functions of the art object in unexpected ways. The power of 'popular art' lies in this synergy, as British anthropologist Karin Barber (1987, p.7) describes: "truly popular art [. . .] is art which furthers the cause of the people by opening their eyes to their objective situation in society. It conscientizes them, thus preparing them to take radical and progressive action".

My working definition of art extends the definition by Fancourt and Finn (2019), to include these contextual African features:

> The art object (whether physical or experiential) is produced through a process requiring novelty, creativity or originality, and specialized skills. It is valued in its own aesthetic right (art for art's sake) and/or as a utility (art for functional use). It provides imaginative experiences for both the producer and (participating) audience, and comprises or provokes emotional, cognitive, physical, social and/or spiritual responses that may drive societal transformation.

The second strand of *Selling Healing* will examine the value of arts applied to health communication interventions. The field of health communication has been described as a transdisciplinary field. Concepts and methods are drawn from the social and health sciences, humanities and arts, "to combine and integrate disciplinary perspectives and build new scientific perspectives and applications" (Kreps and Maibach, 2008, p.732). This transdisciplinary position requires an ecological outlook – an understanding that communication occurs within complex environments and across multiple levels of social organisation. The 'people and places framework' proposed by Edward Maibach and colleagues (2007), who write from a North American perspective, captures the accepted ecological model of health. The framework focuses on three elements:

> (a) the attributes of the people in the population; (b) the attributes of the environments – or places – in which members of the population live, work, go to school, shop and so forth; and (c) important interactions between the attributes of people and places (p.2).

Through levels of analysis or 'fields of influence' these attributes and their interactions "typically influence health through their impact on health behaviour and through direct effects on physical functioning and well-being" (p.2).

Similarly, Campbell and Scott (2011, p.267), writing from the European perspective, list five ways, ranging from the personal to the structural, through which people can be empowered to take control of their health:

> engaging in health-enhancing behaviour change; accessing health services and support; developing health-enabling social capital; engaging in collective action to tackle obstacles to health; and developing health-related social policy (locally, nationally or globally).

Despite a general acceptance of the ecological nature of health and the multi-layered dimensions of health communication, the health communication field – applied across many country settings including Ghana – is dominated by the use of social cognition models. Developed in 'mainstream' health and social psychology, social cognitive models such as the Health Belief Model (HBM) and the Theory of Planned Behaviour (TPB), operate on the assumption that individuals are driven by a common rational desire to preserve health.[17] A typical hypothesis suggests that better individual knowledge and motivational intent will lead to desirable attitudinal and behavioural change. Researchers working from critical disciplinary perspectives argue that this assumption is simplistic. First, an exclusive focus on 'rationality' neglects "'irrational', unconscious forces and emotions" (Crossley, 2000, p.38), which underpin human behaviour. Second, people and places have cultures and histories – therefore health knowledge and behaviours are underpinned, not by a singular rationality but, by multiple rationalities embedded in these cultures and histories. What might be deemed irrational in one setting will be deemed rational in another. Third, people and places are shaped by structured power relations in society that undermine health-enabling behaviours, such as poverty and social isolation. These multilayered factors shape the ways people engage in health-enabling behaviour or in health-damaging behaviour "even when they are in possession of accurate factual information and the resources about health risks and how to avoid them" (Campbell and Scott, 2011, p.267). For example, despite full knowledge of the long-term health-damaging effects of smoking, individuals make a 'rational' choice to smoke as a means of coping with adverse social and material circumstances; or despite full knowledge and understanding of the protective value of condoms, individuals make a 'rational' choice not to use condoms as a

[17] See David Marks (1996) for an early, and still relevant, discussion on the differences between mainstream and critical health psychology.

symbolic and emotional commitment to long-term relationships (Campbell, 2003; Crossley, 2000).

Researchers working at the interface of arts and health communication push these arguments further by considering the multi-layered functions of social memory and social creativity. Brazilian social psychologist Sandra Jovchelovitch (2015), in her work with favela communities in Rio de Janeiro, demonstrates how health knowledge, healing practices and community health development are shaped by 'the creativity of the social': the capacity of individuals and communities 'to imagine alternative possibilities' and to reconfigure current realities and accumulated traditions through 'creative practices of the imagination' in ways that offer healing or catalyse 'social action for change' (p.86). In the first comprehensive scoping review of arts and health promotion in Africa, Christopher Bunn and colleagues (2020) make a similar observation of "the negotiation of social change in Chewa and Manganja communities" in Malawi: "artistic forms and methods facilitate participants to step outside of their everyday lives to use imagination and play to reconfigure how they understand and act on an aspect of life, such as a disease" (p.2). Social creativity during the HIV/AIDS pandemic offers an instructive illustration of how the arts mediate health communication at multiple levels of social organisation and, by extension, expose the limitations of the dominant social cognition models.

During the early decades of the HIV/AIDS pandemic in Africa, the dominant health communication approach was the KAB (knowledge-attitude-behaviour) approach, which was operationalised through the ABC (Abstain Be Faithful use a Condom) message. Across many countries ABC messages created awareness of HIV risks, but awareness did not translate to the desired sexual health protective behaviours (Kalipeni et al., 2004). This social cognition approach failed because it ignored the emotional, social and structural contexts in which intimate relationships operate, such as love, gender and class (Campbell, 2003). Meanwhile, the visceral reality of risk, suffering and loss ignited an explosion of creative responses, particularly in countries hardest hit by the disease, and in countries where political responses were slow and inadequate. In Ethiopia, Ghana, Nigeria, Kenya, Malawi, Morocco, Tanzania, South Africa, Uganda and Zimbabwe, communities responded to HIV/AIDS through song, dance, theatre and comedy (Barz and Cohen, 2011). These creative responses – some new, some reconfigured from local artistic traditions – expanded lay understanding of health promotion imperatives, but also eased the anxieties and stresses brought on by the material and psychological impact of HIV/AIDS. Crucially, communities also engaged in grassroots action, such as lobbying for access to anti-retroviral treatment and social care for families in need. As Thembela Vokwana (2021, p.121) observes, of the South African context, "music performance functioned as a soundtrack in grassroots struggles to anti-retroviral care". In the Ugandan context, ethnomusicologists Gregory Barz and Judah Cohen (2011) observe that 'music as medical intervention' worked in part because "when technical, scientific, or medical 'AIDS talk' was abandoned in favour of 'un-translated' localized terminologies [. . .] audiences appeared much less threatened and anxious (p.8). Heads nod[ded] in agreement or hands clap [ped] in laughter when particular lines resonate[d] with the audience's experience" (p.10). In countries like Uganda, it was the blend of creative expression and empowered action from the grassroots that forced leaders to act on developing and implementing equitable HIV policies. The second strand of the story will track the socio-psychological functions of arts and social creativity in health communication as valuable in and of themselves – for generating well-being, for example – as well as for empowering people to take control over their health in Ghanaian settings.

The final strand of *Selling Healing* will make a case for incorporating arts traditions, whether applied by lay communities or by indigenous healers, into official health communication models and interventions. In African countries, long-standing art traditions intersect with health, illness and healing, such as I have described for Ghanaian communities. Bunn and colleagues (2020, p.2) list five functional applications of the arts in health promotion and argue that these functions "have indigenous roots in African communities":

> creative processes have been harnessed to enquire into local experiences and understandings relating to health, to intervene in drivers of health problems, to provide a discreet form of therapy for a range of conditions and to disseminate and validate health research findings.

A major challenge for arts-based health interventions in African settings is that concepts and methods are driven largely by models developed in the dominant Euro-American arts and health field, which are in turn influenced by culturally specific Euro-American art history and art theory traditions. For example, the Euro-American arts and health field creates distinct categories between art forms: performing *versus* visual *versus* literary arts (Bunn et al., 2020). In contrast, across many African communities, multi-form arts are preferred: performing *and* visual *and* literary arts (Barber, 1987; Ben-Amos, 1989; Bunn et al., 2020). The activation of multiform arts in Ghanaian festivals provides a clear example of this preference. When dominant Euro-American models are applied in African contexts without appropriate cultural grounding, this can lead to poor reception of interventions or negative health outcomes.

Theorists argue that to develop culturally grounded arts-based health interventions in African settings, there has to be a nuanced understanding of what is indigenous to communities and what is alien to them. As Bunn and colleagues (2000, p.11) observe, when an art form that "is assumed to be 'of' a community", such as a traditional dance, is in fact "alien", the art form is treated "as a spectacle and not met with participation".

However, as the preliminary Ghanaian examples show, arts traditions and healing traditions are shaped by strategic cultural borrowing. Jack Goody's (1975, 1987) analysis of knowledge production in LoDagaa (Dagara)[18] communities provides a useful example.[19] Goody observed that knowledge production in LoDagaa was shaped by the interdependency between visible (known, familiar) and invisible (unknown, unfamiliar) worlds. There were three intersecting modes of knowledge and knowledge production tied to distinct social groups: (1) *basic knowledge* drawn from everyday relations and activities, which was the domain of all members of society; (2) *traditional knowledge* drawn from traditional beliefs and myths, which was the domain of traditional leaders and traditional history reciters; and (3) *transformational knowledge* drawn from the invisible world of supernatural "powers, spiritual forces, agencies" (Goody, 1975, p.157), which was the domain of priests, healers and other legitimate social agents with access to the invisible world.

In LoDagaa society, Goody argues, "innovation [was] authorized by outside agencies" (p.165) and religious faith decreed that "in the ambiguity of the creator God [lay] the possibility of change" (p.105). Outside agencies were innovators because they were different and separate from what was known: "they [were] distinct from human society; they [were] importers of new messages, new techniques of the outside world" (p.95). God was powerful precisely because God was ambiguous and unpredictable.

But the psychological draw to the power of outside agencies was also driven by empirical failures in everyday life revealed by basic and traditional knowledge: family relations shifted between strength and fragility,

[18] LoDagaa and Dagara refer to the same ethnic group/community. While scholars like Goody used LoDagaa, the community itself prefers Dagara.

[19] I have drawn on these arguments made by Goody (1975, 1987) and Rekdal (1999) in a conceptual article on knowledge production in African settings (de-Graft Aikins, 2012). I re-present these ideas here, with minor changes.

cults and shrines promised but failed to deliver healing. It is through this tension between the familiar and unfamiliar, that the "process of religious creation [was] rendered almost essential" (Goody, 1987, p.131) and new deities emerged, healers gained their mysterious powers, and cults and shrines proliferated.

Similar phenomena have been reported in medical anthropological studies in other African societies that are "open to the unfamiliar, the alien, the unknown" (Rekdal, 1999, p.458) and for whom, as a consequence, a strong correlation exists between geographical distance and supernatural power. The Norwegian anthropologist Ole Bjørn Rekdal (1999) observed that healing and ritual expertise among the Iraqw people of Tanzania was driven by the "*the power inherent in the ambiguity of the culturally distant*" (p.470, emphasis added). This power operated hand-in-glove with reflexive awareness of weaknesses within Iraqw socio-cultural structures and relationships. At the level of specific groups, there was a tendency for local healers to challenge local political authority in their quest to expand professional expertise. Respect and dissent framed the relationships between healers and political authorities. In broader society, daily social relations were shaped by emotional tensions, such as loyalty and mistrust, based on a reflexive awareness that "the intimacy so highly valued between neighbours render[ed] them vulnerable to each other" (p.468). The complexities of intra-cultural relationships and practices, as well as scepticism about these relationships and practices framed the very nature of cultural openness in Iraqw society. It is within this context, Rekdal argues, that the acceptance of biomedical systems by Iraqw society had to be understood: "biomedicine as a way of understanding and approaching illness was certainly new to the Iraqw; *what was not new was the incorporation of an alien way of looking at and acting on illness*" (p.472, emphasis added). Rekdal speculated that in similarly open African societies, individuals would accept biomedicine, and other foreign medical systems, "precisely because they 'believe in' and 'cling to' their 'native medicine', with its emphasis on the healing power of the culturally distant" (p.473).

In African settings, healing arts, to extend Suzanne Preston Blier's (1993) observation, are grounded in social life. We can argue, therefore, that: (1) in some settings, indigenous arts traditions will have alien elements; and (2) some arts traditions evolve by actively 'incorporating an alien way of looking at' and producing art. Both arguments apply to the production of healing arts in Ghanaian contexts. The stories told and sung by Fante Adzewa groups incorporate cross-cultural elements, borrowed from the Asantes and the English. The lyrics of the ritual songs sung during the Ga Homowo festival blend Ga, Akan, Ewe and English words. Dagomba drums beat Akan proverbs in secular and sacred gatherings. This social psychological character of art production and engagement by lay people and indigenous healers requires systematic analysis in concrete healing contexts. I consider how the arts – whether indigenous, strategically borrowed, or externally imposed – shape representations, imagination, memories, emotions, embodied experiences, relationships and actions along healing journeys across pluralistic healthcare systems.

The Chapters

To understand what works in health communication in Ghanaian contexts, and how creative arts are 'activated' in this sphere, indigenous ways of communicating health and illness and navigating healing journeys have to be understood. In Chapter 2, I will discuss how these dynamics play out in two communities in which I have conducted chronic illness research: Nkoranza, an Akan community in the Bono East (formerly Brong Ahafo) region, and Ga Mashie, a Ga community in the capital Accra. Akan and Ga communities subscribe to a cultural imperative to 'sell one's illness in order to get a cure': "*wo ton wo yareɛ a na wonya n'ano aduro*" (*Twi*); "*ke ohoo ohela, onaa ehe tsofa*" (Ga). The 'selling', I will argue, is health communication. The 'cure' covers a range of therapeutic options including diagnosis, pharmacological, psychological or spiritual treatment, and social advice, support and care. Communities are also hypervigilant about risk in intimate relations, as captured in another proverb: "*Aboa bi reka wo a, öfiri wo ntoma mu*"/ 'if an animal is biting, it is from inside your cloth'. This risk is heightened in contexts of illness and crises. These competing theories complicate the imperative to sell one's sickness. Individuals engage in strategies of partial disclosure and non-disclosure, modulated by levels of trust, especially when illness is chronic or terminal or likely to be stigmatised. Indigenous healers navigate this complicated psychosocial terrain in creative and subversive ways – their goal, to 'sell healing' for all conditions. Signature methods include advertising using multi-form arts, storytelling in diagnostic encounters, and the use of artefacts, costume and performance in healing processes. At the extreme end of this creative enterprise, the category of the 'fake healer' has emerged: a shrine priest, herbalist or pastor whose claims to healing are viewed by society as purely performative and also potentially harmful. I will illustrate where 'selling sickness' meets 're-inventions of healing traditions' in healing environments and healing encounters, and signpost where specific art forms are activated in these spaces.

Colonial era arts-based interventions in the Gold Coast focused on a range of health conditions, including prevalent infectious diseases like malaria and conditions of modernisation such as sexually transmitted diseases in mining towns. I begin Chapter 3 with the example of *Mr Wise and Mr Foolish go to Town*, an ill-conceived educational film on syphilis prevention dispatched from the Colonial Office at Downing Street, London to the Gold Coast Governor's office in Accra in June 1944. This project and other arts-based interventions were embedded in the colonial medicine system which, in turn, was shaped by the 'psychic life of the colonial encounter' (Fanon, 1963): the conditioning of African psychological realities by colonial relations of racialised power, violence and resistance. I contrast the colonial case studies with contemporary global health approaches to arts-based health communication. I argue that the intersection of psychological and political dynamics underpinning encounters between global health actors and local communities, as well as local experts who (claim to) represent, or advocate for, local communities, creates a "psychic life of the global health encounter". This psychic life is also double-edged. When intervention models are imported wholesale into Ghanaian contexts, without cultural grounding and with unexamined prejudices, a range of problems emerge including the imposition of methods and policies that, at best, do not work and, at worst, can cause symbolic and material harm. But in the same way that Ghanaian communities resisted health communication interventions associated with colonial medical violence, communities resist present-day global (arts-based) health interventions that are perceived to be harmful. Strategies of resistance are driven in part by creative practices of the imagination.

Arts-mediated HIV/AIDS education received significant funding from Ghana's donor partners and global health institutions during the first two decades of the pandemic. Yet these interventions had a mixed impact. On the one hand, there was – and continues to be – near universal awareness of HIV/AIDS, including risk factors and health outcomes. On the other hand, low condom use and persistent stigma suggest that knowledge has not translated to sexual health protective behaviours and psychosocial support. In Chapter 4, I will examine how arts were incorporated into HIV/AIDS interventions, focusing on the use of mass media campaigns to raise awareness and educate, and on 'folk media' to educate and empower communities. I discuss a study that applied a narrative approach to examine local knowledge and lived experience – the findings of which illustrate important contrasts between community and indigenous healing system responses to HIV/AIDS and official health service responses. Against the backdrop of recent reports of a resurgence of HIV infections among young Ghanaians, I will end with reflections on what these insights yield for developing more robust arts-based HIV interventions in the future.

In Chapter 5, I focus on the Regenerative Health and Nutrition (RHN) Programme, an intervention that was developed in 2006 by Ghana's Ministry of Health in collaboration with the African Hebrew Development Agency (AHDA), an agency established by a community of African-Americans who had settled in Dimona, Israel and lived a holistic lifestyle. The RHN Programme, piloted in nine districts in the country's (then) ten regions,[20] applied slogans and signposts and the celebrity campaign for its messaging. At its core was the re-imagining of local recipes through the lens of AHDA's trademarked Edenic Divine Diet. While the programme promoted 'food is medicine' through arts-based methods, a competing representation of 'food is poison' prevailed across the RHN communities. This representation, developed from "slow observations" (Davies, 2022) of the "slow violence" (Nixon, 2011) of toxic agricultural practices and environmental degradation, undermined acceptance of the RHN message and intentions to cook and eat more healthily. The arts could not cut through these competing representations. I consider how these broader structural factors interfere with the hybridisation of Ghanaian food cultures and present conceptual challenges for public health nutrition interventions, whether they apply the arts or not.

Ghanaian artist and academic Bernard Akoi-Jackson developed and led a multi-year art therapy programme with patients at Pantang Psychiatric Hospital – one of Ghana's three psychiatric hospitals. Chapter 6 focuses on an exhibition I co-curated with Akoi-Jackson on mental health promotion at the Nubuke Foundation, Accra, in 2009, that was inspired by this programme. Sketches, paintings, screen prints, and fabric work produced by patients were exhibited alongside commissioned paintings on a predetermined theme of 'mental health' from established Ghanaian contemporary artists and photographs from an anthropological study on mental healthcare in shrines and prayer camps conducted by British anthropologist Ursula Read. Through a photo story approach, I detail the rationale and process of curating the exhibition and discuss visitors' responses,

[20] The ten regions were re-zoned to sixteen regions in 2020, after a referendum held in 2018 with targeted districts resulted in a 99 per cent yes vote. See Map in Appendix 1.

which converged on two themes: the art exhibition as a viable approach for mental health promotion; and arts therapies as methods of rehumanising the psychiatric space. I reflect on the curating process and what this revealed about the multi-layered challenges that face individuals and families affected by severe chronic mental illness and where the arts can play a role in forging more robust collaborations between psychiatric and indigenous healing systems.

In 2019, the NCD Alliance – the global civil society network dedicated to noncommunicable diseases (NCD) advocacy – developed a project called *Our Views, Our Voices*. Training on NCD storytelling was organised in a number of countries including Ghana, with the aim to "enable individuals living with NCDs to share their views to take action and drive change". The local Ghanaian advert called for English speakers (only) to apply for limited spaces for training. My research team applied for two members of Jamestown Health Club – a patient support group based in Ga Mashie – to participate in the training. Their analysis of the workshop was captured in a rhetorical question: "we tell the stories – and then what? We cannot eat the stories". In Chapter 7, I examine the encounter between the NCD Alliance storytelling project and the local patient advocacy movement and discuss the scope and limits of storytelling for 'taking action and driving change' for NCD prevention and control in Ghana. I argue that the NCD Alliance project builds on a chequered history of global health storytelling, such as the HIV confessional technology (Nguyen, 2010), where cultural appropriation meets corporate branding. Narrative is central to social life, and stories of lived experiences of illness have reported benefits, including for educating communities at risk, and facilitating coping and conscientisation in patient groups. But the culture and politics of storytelling also matter: in Ghanaian communities affected by chronic conditions, careful considerations are made about why a story must be told in the first place, who to tell the story to, and when, where and how to tell the story. Crucially, investing in narrative health at the expense of structural and political solutions to complex health problems can have harmful consequences, particularly for marginalised communities.

During the first year of the global COVID-19 pandemic, Ghana's creative arts communities captured its complex facets through various art forms. In Chapter 8, I focus on how these spontaneous artistic responses afforded the opportunity to examine in real time how grassroots arts and bottom-up social responses to health crises influenced health communication. Working with a local team, I tracked and collated various art forms of this genre of 'COVID arts' including comedy sketches, cartoons, songs, textile designs and murals. I outline the methods used to define and track COVID-19 arts, detail their communicative functions, and reflect on insights these new art forms present for pandemic health communication. Artists channelled 'creative practices of the imagination' regarding COVID-19, highlighting a mutually constitutive relationship between lay responses to the pandemic and what artists produced. The COVID arts they produced functioned in three arts and health domains: health education and knowledge production, disease prevention, and (indirectly) COVID-19 policy development. These intersecting functions converged on the science, culture and politics of COVID-19. I will outline the subtle and radical ways artists translated the science, culture and politics of the COVID-19 pandemic to Ghanaian communities at home and abroad. I reflect on the insights these new art forms present for health communication during the COVID-19 pandemic and beyond.

In the concluding Chapter 9, I return to the three narrative strands of *Selling Healing* through a synthesis of cross-cutting themes emerging from the case studies. I explore the possibilities of operationalising the Akan concept of Sankofa for indigenising health communication models. Sankofa means 'to retrieve'. The concept is captured in the proverb: "*Se wo were fi na wosan kofa a yenkyiri*" / 'It is not taboo to fetch what is at risk of being left behind' (Appiah et al., 2008). It is also represented visually, in gold weights, wood sculptures and textile designs by a bird that moves forward while turning its head back (see Frontispiece). Sankofa has become an organising interdisciplinary principle for developing a decolonial *and* indigenising approach to identity, agency, and social change for continental and diaspora African communities (Matemba, 2020; Pence et al., 2023). I define Sankofa from a social psychological perspective, as a creative practice of the imagination and memory – a vital process of remembering and reclaiming lost or contested traditions within the boundaries of self, society and culture and activating these traditions to serve contemporary needs.

CHAPTER 2

If You Sell Your Sickness You Get a Cure

Wo ton wo yareɛ a na wonya n'ano aduro | If you sell your sickness, you get a cure

Aboa bi reka wo a, öfiri wo ntoma mu | if an animal is biting, it is from inside your cloth

Akan proverbs[1]

Selling Sickness: Ruth's Story

In 2001, I interviewed Ruth, a woman in her 50s, who lived in Nkoranza in the Bono East Region. Ruth lived with type 2 diabetes and was one of several adult men and women I interviewed for my doctoral research on the social representations of diabetes in Nkoranza, the neighbouring Kintampo, as well as in Accra and Tema.[2] Ruth attributed her diabetes to her unhealthy lifestyle. She described herself as a woman who loved the high life when she was younger. As a successful trader, she made enough money to indulge in sweet foods, as well as alcohol and cigarettes. But she also suspected, following a casual comment made by an acquaintance, that she might have got diabetes through her brother's sorcery.

RUTH: [. . .] a certain woman came here to work. She worked with my brother. One day, she and my brother had a quarrel. In the course of the quarrel, she told my brother 'You have bought disease for your sister'. This is what the woman told my brother.

[1] All Akan proverbs in *Selling Healing* are taken from a compilation of 7,015 proverbs by Peggy Appiah, Kwame Anthony Appiah and Ivor Agyemang-Duah (2008). The authors offer the literal English translation, followed by the proverb's deeper meaning. For example, the second proverb means "a person close to you is the most likely to harm you" (p.186).

[2] de-Graft Aikins (2005). All participant names are anonymised, except in cases where permission has been granted for real names to be used (see, e.g., Chapter 7).

DANSO YEBOAH[3] (DY, interviewing): You mean the woman said this to your brother?

RUTH: After the woman has said this, I said, 'oh, brother, thank you for doing this to me'. My brother did not say a word.

DY: In your own view, what do you really think brings about this diabetes disease?

RUTH: I do ask, whether it is because of the sugar I eat or what? As for me, I really like sugar.

DY: Does that make you think that (you got diabetes) because of the sugar that you eat?

RUTH: For me, what I think could be the cause, is my brother.

Ruth received treatment from St Theresa's Hospital, Nkoranza's sole government hospital. She also sought faith healing through all-night prayer sessions at her local church, and experimented with home remedies and herbal supplements recommended by friends and acquaintances. But she could not afford the prescribed insulin, her diabetes was poorly managed as a result, and she had lost a considerable amount of weight. Her daughter and primary caregiver, Adjoa, observed: "In fact, we were all shocked to see how a fat woman like her would reduce in size like that."

In Nkoranza in the 1990s and early 2000s, as was the case across many African communities, rapid and sustained weight loss was associated with HIV/AIDS. Ruth experienced HIV-related stigma from the community. As her health waned, she had downsized her trading activities for food hawking – she made 'rice water' (rice porridge) for sale in the mornings. When she began losing weight, rumours and gossip led to former friends and acquaintances shunning her. She lost customers.

> When I sent food to the school to sell, the children wouldn't buy the food, because the teacher told them I have HIV/AIDS.

Her family lived with "courtesy stigma" (Goffman, 1963/1990). Adjoa's attempt to take over her mother's food hawking business failed because people were unwilling to buy food from an individual living in close proximity to an alleged AIDS sufferer.

> You see, at first, my mother was selling rice water. Due to her illness I had to take over and sell it but people didn't buy it anymore. Some people thought she had got AIDS. This perception hung over her and made people stop buying her rice water.

[3] Danso Yeboah, a research staff member at Kintampo Health Research Centre, provided Twi interviewing assistance for my data collection in Kintampo and Nkoranza.

American sociologist Kathy Charmaz (1983) proposed the concept of 'loss of self' to describe 'a fundamental form of suffering' for people living with debilitating chronic illness. 'Loss of self' occurred at four intersecting socio-psychological levels: living a restricted life, existing in social isolation, experiencing discredited definitions of self, and harbouring a fear of becoming a burden to significant others. Ruth experienced these four levels of loss of self due to the disruptive medical, financial, social and psychological impact of diabetes.

Her relationship with her daughter and other family members suffered. Daily interactions were characterised by emotional tensions due to misunderstandings, mistrust, fear and physical exhaustion.

RUTH: I gave birth to twelve children, but there are only nine left. [. . .]. Those that are with me here are not responsible for my living. When they cook they don't even give me some to eat. They claim I am a witch. As a result they don't even give me food to eat.

ADJOA: If I have, I give her. If I don't have too, I make her aware that I don't have it. I am under pressure. I have realized that in Nkoranza if you have no one to help you in times of trouble, you worry a lot. When the impact of the disease increases, I feel a lot of pressure. She worries me a lot and so I make up my mind to travel and leave her, if we leave and later we hear that she is dead, then we can come back and bury her. But I have second thoughts and then decide to stay and take care of her.

Ruth belonged to a diabetes self-help group established by a senior nurse at St Theresa's Hospital. Several other members of the group experienced loss of self, but to a lesser degree. As one member observed of Ruth's circumstances: "[W]e are all suffering, but hers is extreme."

Ruth was not the only person who attributed her type 2 diabetes to a blend of natural, social and supernatural factors – a good proportion of self-help group members reported eclectic diabetes causal theories. These shared theories aligned with what has been termed the tripartite model of African health beliefs. The model has three elements. In *Traditional Medical Systems of Ghana*, the Ghanaian medical sociologist Patrick A. Twumasi (1975) referred to these elements, in the Akan context, as physically caused conditions (*ho nam mu yadee*), economically or socially oriented conditions (*asetana mu nsem*) and spiritually caused conditions (*sunsum mu yadee*).[4] Physically caused conditions (*ho nam mu yadee*) occurred through natural elements such as heat, cold, injuries and pollution and included malaria, fevers and general aches and pains. Socially

[4] For Ga communities, see Field (1937) and Mullings (1984).

caused conditions (*asetana mu asem*) occurred through the "conscious or unconscious interpersonal malevolence" (Helman, 2000, p.93) characteristic of witchcraft and sorcery.[5] Spiritually caused conditions (*sunsum yadee*) were caused through the direct action of God (the Supreme Being), lesser gods and ancestral spirits. Rare or unnatural events such as the death of a child or young adult, chronic physical and mental illnesses, or illnesses that caused sudden death in otherwise healthy adults were attributed to social and/or spiritual causes.

Decision-making on healthcare was typically facilitated by a "therapy managing group" (Janzen, 1978): "[T]he family support system for sick individuals that made decisions at every stage of the disease course, even though they had no specialized knowledge of disease or therapy." The therapeutic journey is often a shared journey between individuals living with illness and their caregivers. The cognitive, emotional and spiritual resources that are drawn on to address the effects of illness in the short or long term are often shared resources. However, when individuals live with *sunsum mu yadee* or *asetena mu yadee*, family members are often viewed as conduits of these conditions. Ruth's reference to a "bought disease" (*nto yare*, Twi) describes conditions that arise from psychospiritual factors such as sorcery and witchcraft and are rooted in toxic interpersonal and social relationships and corrosive emotions, such as envy, jealousy and hatred. These psychospiritual drivers of illness and misfortune are anticipated in daily life. Proverbs warn of risk in intimate relationships: "*Aboa bi reka wo a, ɔ̈firi wo ntoma mu*"/'if an animal is biting, it is from inside your cloth'. Research suggests hypervigilance of the "dark side of kinship" (Geschiere, 2003) or "enemyship" ("a form of personal relationship involving hatred, malice, and sabotage" (Adams and Dzokoto, 2003, p.346) across many social groups. Therapy managing roles within the family are complicated by these representations. For Ruth and her family, and for families who made sense of diabetes through the lens of *nto yare*, family members were not viewed as important 'therapy managers' but as *therapy damagers*: people 'with bad minds' or 'dark spirits' who set out to forestall or damage effective therapies.

Nkoranza's healthcare system was pluralistic. In addition to St Theresa's Hospital, there were local pharmacies and licensed chemical sellers. There was a collection of herbalists and shrine priests, whose distinct areas of expertise mapped onto the four Akwapim healer categories delineated by Mohr (2009) (Chapter 1): priests (*asofo*), prophets (*akomfo*), medicine

[5] Helman (2000, p.93).

makers (*aduruyefo*) and herbalists (*adunsifo*). There were churches representing orthodox (e.g., Methodist) and Pentecostal denominations. The Pentecostal churches operated prayer camps that offered healing for a variety of health conditions, including diabetes and mental illness.

Within this pluralistic medical system, shrine priests and herbalists wielded power in the domain of sicknesses that had ambiguous roots and manifestations. They operated in the liminal space between the cultural imperative to sell sickness on the one hand and, on the other hand, fear-driven hypervigilance about 'the dark side of kinship'. They understood the complicated emotions driving personal, interpersonal and group relations and the fundamental need to domesticate the symbolic and concrete threats posed by protracted illness. They also followed national biomedical discourse on public health trends to identify new conditions that could expand their open-ended list of curable diseases. It is in this dynamic epidemiological space that their power had always emerged and where strategies of creative borrowing operated. Even their professional rivals knew this. An endocrinologist I interviewed in Accra, in 2001, observed:

> The traditional healers do not advertise treatment for hypercholesterolemia. Yeah they don't advertise treatment for hypercholesterolemia for the simple reason that they don't hear a lot spoken about it. But let me get up today and get on the air and let me sort of set up an association for lipid disorders and so on and so forth and the traditional healers will find a remedy for it and say that it is curable.[6]

In Nkoranza, lay and professional groups attributed spiritual causes to chronic conditions and believed shrines and Christian faith healers were experts in diagnosis and treatment. The spiritual elements invariably involved therapy damagers (family witches and sorcerers) or supernatural forces (the devil, evil spirits, God and lesser gods).

> Young woman: "I didn't know it was that disease [*diabetes*] so I went – the doctor examined me and saw nothing. One nurse told me that my sickness must be *abonsam yare* (devil's illness) and that I should go home and find another means of cure. I became so frightened."

Professional groups emphasised their unique ability to address the spiritual roots of health conditions. In their assessment, biomedical professionals lacked this ability. But, they did not only pit this unique expertise against the perceived limitations of biomedicine; they also competed against each

[6] de-Graft Aikins (2005, p.298).

other, making distinctions between nuanced treatment approaches required to counter different categories of spirits and supernatural forces.

FAITH HEALER: "In cases of infertility for example a women might be sent to a doctor but as the doctor works on the problem we pray for the woman, as they work, we work."

SHRINE PRIEST: "When you are tortured spiritually by *abosom* [deities], then it means they want you to tell the truth, they do not want to kill you. So if you go to hospital and you are not conscious of it, the doctor will try as much as he can to no avail. There are others who are tortured by *abosom*, who then take refuge in the church and continually worry the doctors instead of asking for our help.

Lay people understood the technical limits of each system and made strategic choices to avoid harmful services. For practising Christians, the harms posed by shrines appeared to be rooted in their unchecked spiritual power.

ELDERLY MAN: I've been for prayers before. That caused my leg to be amputated. When my leg started, I went to the hospital several times. Now everyone said my disease was demonic so I should go for prayers. I went to Goka[7] and spent 3 months there. Then my leg began to rot. No medicine was applied there. It was just prayer and fasting. I could not sleep at night."

AKOSUA (IN A GROUP DISCUSSION WITH YOUNG PEOPLE): "Please, with *ebibiduro* [literally, Black people's or African medicine, in Twi] those who give you the drugs, *edunsifoo* [shrine priests] if you go there for treatment, they can tell you to bring a chicken, or bring this amount of money, or kneel in front of the shrine, to receive the medication. Perhaps you are a Christian, trying out this treatment, being made to do things which I *feel* you might be uncomfortable doing. So I feel that with ethnomedicine, sometimes you get to the point where going to these kinds of places might not be a good idea."

KOFI (TO SOME LAUGHTER IN THE GROUP): "It isn't good, don't say it might not be good."

In constructing representations of diabetes, people in Nkoranza drew on different systems of knowledge – some complementary, some contradictory – in terms of the relationship and relevance of diabetes to their personal and professional lives.

The concept of 'cognitive polyphasia' was proposed by French social psychologist Serge Mosocovi (2008, p.245) to describe the "tendency to employ diverse and even opposite ways of thinking" when groups and

[7] Goka, a town in the Bono East region, has a famous Pentecostal Christian prayer camp.

individuals are faced with unfamiliar phenomena or 'familiar alien threats'.[8] Moscovici (2008, p.245) argued that this tendency "is a normal state of affairs in ordinary life and communication". In the multidisciplinary literature on illness representations and experiences, several studies report meaning-making as cognitive polyphasic processes (see, e.g., de-Graft Aikins et al., 2023; Marshall et al., 2012). In some circumstances, holding inconsistent ideas or beliefs or expressing inconsistent behaviours can lead to psychological tension or discomfort ('cognitive dissonance'), as when Akosua expressed her views on Christians seeking treatment from shrine priests. In other circumstances, individuals can hold inconsistent or oppositional ideas and engage in contradictory behaviours with no psychological discomfort, as when Ruth made sense of her diabetes through sugar and witchcraft theories and sought biomedical, ethnomedical and faith healing.[9]

As we will see in later sections and subsequent chapters, these complicated thinking-feeling processes inform lay understandings of health conditions and shape healthcare behaviours across several Ghanaian communities. Cognitive polyphasia fixes attention to cultural modes of health knowledge production (e.g., the tripartite model) but also reveals the ways everyday knowledge production, through a rootedness in embodied experiences and social relations, transcends culture. Examining meaning-making through this social psychological framework facilitates a conceptual openness to locally situated ways of being, knowing, feeling and acting in relation to health, illness and healing. And since the arts are "grounded in social life" (Blier, 1993), this framework also facilitates conceptual tracking of the way arts and social creativity function as knowledge systems in health communication.

Selling Healing: Shrine Priests and Herbalists

In the 1980s, African-American sociologist Leith Mullings (1984) conducted ethnographic research on mental health and healing in Labadi, an

[8] Social psychologists define familiar alien threats as 'categories of phenomena or people, like madness or the mentally ill, that we may already know but actively "maintain in an unfamiliar position", because they represent danger, chaos, or transgression' (de-Graft Aikins, 2020, p.403 referencing Kalampalikis and Haas, 2008 and Rose, 1998).

[9] Marshall et al. (2012) conducted a systematic review of qualitative research on lay perspectives on hypertension and drug adherence in sixteen countries across Africa, Asia, Australia, Europe, North America and South America. They reported that, across settings, individuals drew on eclectic sources of knowledge to make sense of hypertension; they "often held mutually contradictory explanations, and the inconsistencies did not trouble them" (p.5).

indigenous Ga community in Accra. She observed adults and children who sought diagnosis and treatment from herbalists, pastors and shrine priests for various mental health problems: depression, anxiety, night terrors and psychosis.

Mullings documented the way shrine priests diagnosed and treated presenting health conditions through the use of "social facts" – which she defined as "views, grievances, feelings, attitudes held by various individuals in different structural positions, in relation to a specific case at hand" (p.81). These social facts were woven into diagnostic encounters in creative ways, through suggestion, storytelling and the deployment of ritual objects. "Much of healing", Mullings (1984, p.56) observed, "was art, involving the idiosyncratic".

One of the cases Mullings observed involved a young woman called Aba who, with the help of her mother, sought diagnosis and treatment from a prominent traditional healer, Ataa, after experiencing mental health distress. Ataa was the second stop along a healer-shopping journey. The first stop had been a spiritualist church, which had not provided the absolute healing required.

Mullings reports:

> Early one morning in the beginning of October, Aba arrived at the healer's compound accompanied by her mother and her mother's sister's daughter. [...] The three women, the healer, and his eldest wife (Aba's mother's sister) entered the inner room for the divination procedure. Needless to say, the social facts of the case were well known to the healer through his wife. First the healer wrote their family names and day names on a piece of paper in which he wrapped two cedis in silver coins. He placed this package under an old broken mirror to which was attached a bone. Aba directed her soliloquy to the healer. [...]. The healer then poured schnapps over the mirror and the various representations of the gods (*wokui*). Lighting a candle, he passed over the mirror with a circular motion seven times. He threw six cowrie shells onto the back of the mirror, observing the pattern in which they fell. After pouring libation for the gods housed separately in a smaller room, he threw the cowrie shells a second time. In reaction to the healer shaking his head and kissing his teeth after a second glimpse into the mirror, Aba began to talk compulsively again. [...] Although Aba was a practising Christian, she called on the spirits of the healer's medicines, the town gods ancestral shades as well as Nyongmo (God), to help her (Mullings, 1984, pp.84–87).

The consultation lasted three hours and ended with Ataa diagnosing "a spiritual illness" and presenting a list of fourteen items Aba and her mother were required to bring the following day to begin treatment.

> 1 bottle of palm oil, a pure black fowl, 77 red kola nuts, 1 bottle of schnapps, 9 eggs ('the good ones, not the ones that come from the poultry farm'), one box of powder, 12 yards of white calico, 12 yards of dark blue calico, 1 packet of candles, 7 crabs, 1 cigarette tin of small red peppers, 1 bunch of small onions, 1 cigarette tin of salt, I large bowl for mashing the small peppers (Mullings, 1984, p.87).

In Mullings' ethnographic description, prior knowledge of the social facts of Aba's case and the use of objects, symbols and performance were central to diagnosis and treatment. Aba's mother's sister was married to Ataa. The social facts of Aba's case were therefore closer to hand compared to usual cases.

The bone, the representation of the gods (*wokui*) and cowrie shells created an atmosphere drenched with ritual symbolism. Similarly, particular items on the treatment list – palm oil, schnapps, white and blue calico – had symbolic value and function (Akyeampong, 1995; Breidenbach, 1976). For instance, Ghanaian historian Emmanuel Akyeampong (1995, p.266) notes that alcohol is a "ritual artifact" for Akan, Ga-Adangme, Ewe and Dagaba communities because it "facilitate[s] communication between the spiritual and physical worlds".[10] The list also blended the old and new, familiar and imported items from other ethnic healing traditions and farther afield: kola nuts (typically used in northern healing repertoires), schnapps and the cigarette tin (likely European).

Aba and her mother brought the prescribed items to begin treatment. The process took three months and involved "medications, baths, sacrifices and special rituals" (Mullings, 1984, p.92). It was an unpredictable and psychologically draining journey for Aba and her family. By January of the following year, where Mullings ended the story, Aba had not received the healing she desired.

In 2018, I interviewed Nai Wulomo, the Chief Priest of Ga Mashie, as part of my long-term social psychological study of chronic illness and care in the community (de-Graft Aikins et al., 2020). Situated a few miles to the west of Labadi, Ga Mashie is a township of two communities, Jamestown and Usshertown. Like Labadi and other Ga communities situated along Ghana's coast, Ga Mashie lived through imperial trade, slavery, colonialism and the establishment of Accra as the capital of the Gold Coast in 1877. A history of urbanisation, globalisation and multi-culture in Ga Mashie has

[10] Akyeampong (1995) notes that "male elders in pre-colonial southern Ghana viewed drink as possessing potent spiritual power; without drink, one could not communicate through libation (Twi: *nsa guo or mpae yi*) with the ancestors and the gods" (p.266). Libation was central to a broad range of social events: rites of passage, festivals, child naming, marriages and funerals.

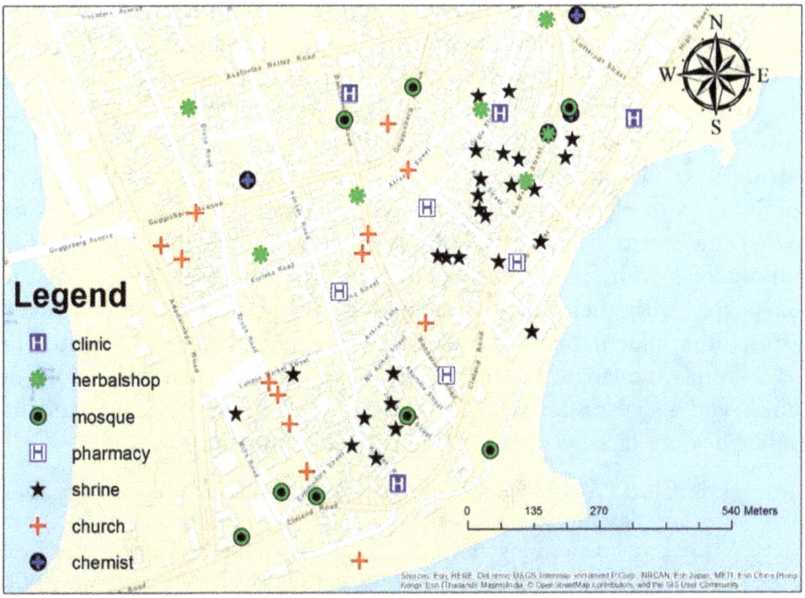

Figure 2.1 Pluralistic healthcare facilities in Ga Mashie in 2014.

forged a dynamic hybrid space that blends the old and new, the familiar and strange (Akyeampong, 2002; Robertson, 1984). The community's pluralistic healthcare system captures this hybridity. Previously, my team had mapped out the spatial organisation of healthcare services in the community (Figure 2.1). Of the sixty healthcare facilities in the community, almost half were traditional shrines (twenty-seven): the rest were one government polyclinic, three private clinics, four private pharmacies, three licensed chemical sellers, thirteen churches and eight mosques.

The traditional shrines in Ga Mashie are dominant, not only in number but also in their spiritual power (Field, 1937; Mullings, 1984). These shrines were present in the community long before the arrival of Christian missionaries and churches and before colonial biomedical facilities were built. Korle-Bu Teaching Hospital, the country's premier teaching hospital, situated in the Korle Gonno suburb a few miles to the west of Ga Mashie, was built in 1924. Shrines were the preferred source for addressing social and psychological problems.[11] The Chief Priest presided over these shrines and the

[11] This was an accepted fact, even by Christian ministers serving the community, according to a 2015 interview I conducted with a local Presbyterian minister.

shrine priests and priestesses, providing spiritual and institutional guidance, as well as forging links with the broader Ga political system.

Nai Wulomo welcomed us with his support team of male healers and elders. His description of his healing repertoire was intertwined with the history of pre-colonial, colonial and contemporary Ga communities. His historical knowledge was drawn from eclectic sources, part factual, part mythical, with elements drawn from the "Klama", a 400-year-old song cycle sung in part at the annual Homowo festival.[12] He mixed Ga healing philosophies with Bible verses, juxtaposed the migration history of the Ga people with their colonial encounter with Europeans. He invoked nature, the supernatural and social relations as drivers of diseases in Ga Mashie. Similar to Ataa in 1980s Labadi, the spiritual dimensions of illness and social crises were key to the Chief Priest's practice, and he gathered social facts to inform diagnosis and treatment.

> As the Chief Priest I have the authority. We are consulted when it is realized that the sickness is spiritual then I will perform a ritual to reverse the curse. When I am performing the ritual [...] the number of herbs used will depend on the day of the week and the day on which the person was born. We count till 7 and fetch the sea water. We then add rain water and what the Christians call Holy Water. We then bathe you with the mixture. We add palm [oil] to drive the evil spirit. Whatever is done with liquor cannot be replaced with water. In the olden days, they were using alcohol and that is what we have been introduced to so we have been using Schnapps. When I wake up, I will pray for the entire community and when it is 6 o'clock, I will drive away all the evil forces. I will stand at the various 7 streets and junctions [...] and drive away the evil forces and if any negative thing has been spoken against us, I will reverse this.

Healing was a collaborative practice. Each member of his healing team had unique skills for pivotal points along the healing journey. He pointed to a young man who sat among the elders on the bench in front of us. This young man, he informed us, had been born with a gift of 'spiritual sight'. He had the ability to see the invisible, the not-yet-known. Spiritual sight was crucial to diagnosing and treating conditions with spiritual dimensions.

> whatever sickness that can be seen in the physical can also be done in the spiritual/ caused spiritually. Every sickness can be done in the spirit and that

12 Victoria Ellen Smith (2018) describes the Klama as "an astonishing song cycle, which consists of upwards of 60,000 stanzas, kept by heart for over four hundred years, and sung, in part, at every festival" (p.139). See also historian Irene Odotei's (2016) observation of the La community's version.

> can only be seen by those with spiritual eyes. This can be reversed in the spirit or paid in the spirit to regain the health of the affected person. This is done through a small ritual. The ritual can be done by only those with spiritual eyes; those who can see in the spirit. Like the physical ones that doctors treat, when the spiritual cause is identified, then it is treated. The herbs that you see over there individually have their own uses – what they cure and the combinations of herbs that can cure certain ailments.

With the exception of the herbs the Chief Priest pointed out, the room in which my team and I were received did not have the healing paraphernalia documented in Ataa's room: there was no mirror, representation of the gods (*wokui*), bones or cowrie shells. This was a modern space with a laptop on a table in one corner and, in the opposite corner, a television tuned into an international football game. The Chief Priest had a Public Relations Officer – a young man who facilitated our Saturday afternoon meeting and referred to himself as the 'PRO'. But art and everyday objects "loaded with spiritual power" (Ba, 1976; Leyten, 2015) were strategically placed in the compound and woven into our encounter that afternoon. A bundle of long sticks secured by iron clamps on the ground, called 'pampi', lay at the entry gate of the compound, behind which footwear had to be placed (Figure 2.2).[13] A calabash of water was passed round the room for each person to take a sip as greetings were exchanged.[14] A mural on the wall opposite our meeting room captured, in image and text, aspects of the origin story we had just been told (Figure 2.3): a black Ga hand (likely a traditional leader or healer, based on the white bead bracelet around the wrist) shaking a white European hand (likely a colonial administrator, based on the suit cuffs); the backdrop of huts on land versus one ship on the ocean; the oar versus the broom (a symbol of cleansing); the Ga phrase 'shikpon nεε ononi' and the declaration of cultural and ritual power over space and time in the captions "Acknowledged as King of Akra" and "AD1000". A local artist, Attaa Koblah, was commissioned to paint the mural in 2016.[15]

[13] 'Pampi' – also known as Asoplo sticks (*Asoplo Tsee*) or stone sticks (*Te Tsee*) – is a clear example of an everyday object "loaded with spiritual power" (Ba, 1976). In a follow-up interview with the Chief Priest's PRO (Leslie Mills Lamptey) in March 2024, he observed that pampi "indicates that the house you are entering is not a small house. And if you have a bad mind or bad ideas in your head, you cannot enter or be inside the house. If you try and enter what is in your mind will vanish or you will not remember it."

[14] Like the bundle of sticks, the calabash is an everyday object – used to serve water or drinks in homes, local bars and restaurants. But the calabash also serves ritual purposes in cultural ceremonies and in healing spaces, for example, as a container for medicine (Leyten, 2015).

[15] Interview with the Chief Priest, March 2024. The mural presented here was painted over in 2020 by another commissioned artist called Sodjah. New visual features (such as a gong gong

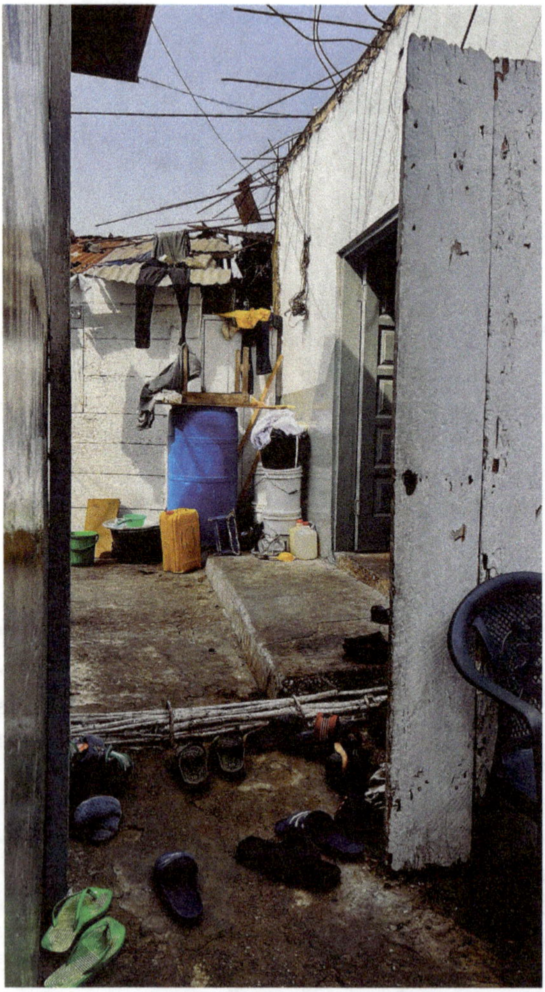

Figure 2.2 Pampi at the entry gate of the Ga Mashie Chief Priest's compound.

The Chief Priest wore the white traditional attire and headdress of shrine priests, accessorised with white bead bracelets on both wrists and left ankle, and a white bead necklace – marking the formality of our meeting (Figure 2.4). His team wore ordinary everyday clothes.

and a row of pots leading to one hut) were incorporated into the 2020 mural to explain, more clearly, the cultural and historical healing in Ga Mashie. See Appendix 3a for the new mural and the symbolic features described by the Chief Priest.

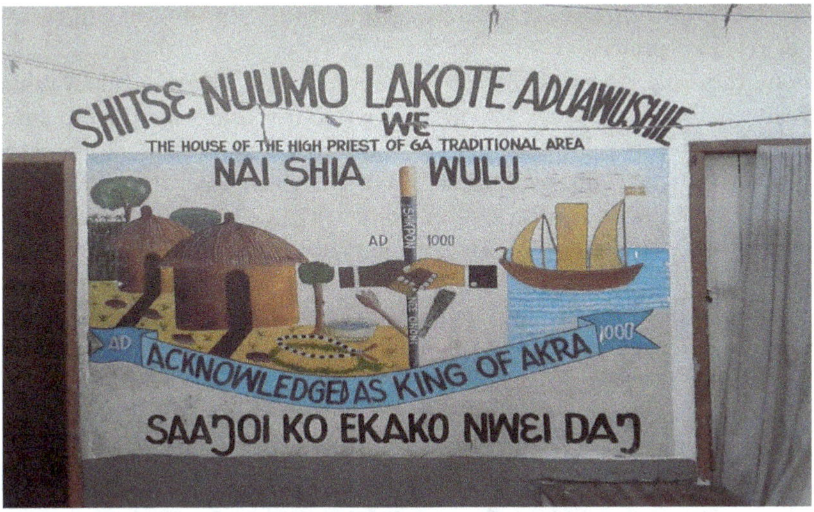
SHITSƐ NUUMO LAKOTE ADUAWUSHIE
WE
THE HOUSE OF THE HIGH PRIEST OF GA TRADITIONAL AREA
NAI SHIA WULU
AD 1000
AD ACKNOWLEDGED AS KING OF AKRA 1000
SAAŊOI KO EKAKO NWƐI DAŊ

Figure 2.3 Mural on the wall of the Ga Mashie Chief Priest's compound.

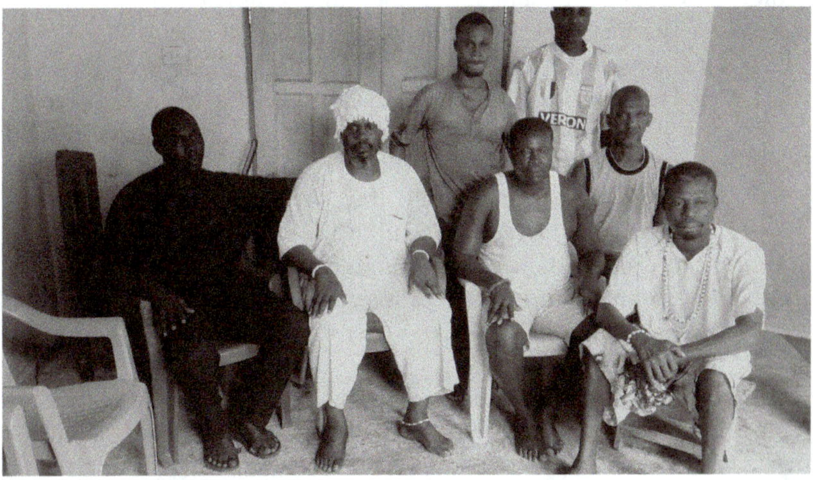

Figure 2.4 Ga Mashie Chief Priest and his team.

In the past, shrine priests like Ataa and Nai Wulomo were found by word of mouth and through their physical presence in their communities. Their pivotal role during annual festivals also opened them up to new clients.[16] Now, there are innovations in advertising the services of indigenous religious healers.

In the early 2000s, a flamboyant shrine priest called Nana Kwaku Bonsam (Bonsam means 'devil' in Twi) burst into Ghanaian public consciousness. His introduction came through a public fight he started with charismatic Pentecostal priests in Ghana, which was avidly covered by the Ghanaian news media. Kwaku Bonsam claimed that the Pentecostal priests had acquired their congregations through spiritual powers he bestowed upon them for a fee. Having achieved their desired congregant numbers, they had reneged on paying for Bonsam's service. Kwaku Bonsam circulated a mythical origin story of his healing gift. In 1992, at age 19, he suffered severe life-altering injuries during a gas explosion. Following his miraculous recovery, he experienced a spiritual transformation, renounced his membership of the Seventh-Day Adventist Church, changed his name (from Stephen Osei Mensah) and established his shrine, which he named Kofioo Kofi. In a short period of time, Nana Kwaku Bonsam built a global brand across the Ghanaian and African diaspora, aided by his larger-than-life personality, a website and social media accounts. Among many strategic claims aimed at amplifying his global brand, he claimed he caused the knee injury suffered by Portuguese footballer Cristiano Ronaldo during the 2014 World Cup.[17] His aim in going global was to spread the gospel of African Traditional Religion, which he believed was more spiritually powerful than Pentecostal Christianity. His global clientele flew him to their cities in Europe and North America, hosted him in their living rooms and generated frenzied fan clubs with branded paraphernalia. In 2013, he spent a year in New York to receive medical treatment, but he also paid for media advertising targeting the diaspora Ghanaian community and held consultations for clients in his Bronx apartment. He was featured in The New York Times, by American journalist Jed Lipinski, under the headline: "A visit from the devil."[18]

More recently, Kwaku Bonsam's marketing success has been eclipsed by the public performances of Nana Agradaa (Patricia Asiedu), a former shrine priestess turned Christian prophetess. Nana Agradaa made a public declaration of her conversion from traditional religion to Christianity on social media and promptly went viral. She then transformed her thriving

[16] Odotei (2016); Parker (2000).
[17] "Ghanaian witch doctor claims he caused Cristiano Ronaldo's knee injury" | The Guardian.
[18] Lipinki (2013).

shrine practice into a Charismatic Pentecostal Church called Heaven Way Champions International Ministry. She established two television stations – Thunder TV and Ice TV – allegedly without licences and built a social media following on TikTok and YouTube. The church swiftly gathered congregants in the thousands through her multi-pronged media advertising. In 2022, Nana Agradaa was arrested and arraigned in court over a financial scam called 'sika garri' (garri money), in which she claimed she could double financial investments for her congregants.[19] Investors did not receive the promised interest or their initial capital. Nana Agradaa mounted a robust defence of herself on social media and was supported by her congregation, her adult son and several fans who have cheered her on since her public debut as a reformed shrine priestess. Her daily social media posts continue to ignite viral conversations, cultivate new followers and generate revenue. In keeping with the importance of hybrid identities for Pentecostal and other Evangelical Christian leaders, Nana Agradaa now refers to herself – and insists on being referred to – as "Reverend Dr Prophetess Evangelist Mama Pat".[20]

Leith Mullings described traditional Ga medicine, *tsofa*, as being both "symbolic and physiological", "sacred and mundane", "visible and invisible" (Mullings, 1984, pp.94–95). Contemporary shrine priests embody these characteristics in public and in spectacular ways. What they do is nothing new, however. In nineteenth-century Akwapim towns, shrine priests experimented with hyphenated identities (Mohr, 2009). Shrines in these towns – such as Akonedi in Larteh – that trace their lineage over centuries remain powerful today. Decades before Kwaku Bonsam held court in the Bronx, Mullings (1984) recalls a 'sherry party' she attended in New York in the 1970s which had been thrown to welcome a famous Akonedi shrine priestess after her successful tour of the United States: the tour had been sponsored by 'a group of Afro-Americans'. "Chiefs, lawyers, doctors, politicians and other notable dignitaries attended the gathering; many greeted her in a way that accorded her more status than several of the chiefs" (p.40). The Akonedi shrine remains powerful not only for clients from all over the country seeking solutions to health and social problems, but also for healers in the African diaspora seeking a stamp of authentic indigenous healing expertise (Guedj, 2015).

19 Garri is a grain made from dried grated cassava. When dry, it resembles couscous. Its key feature is that it expands in volume when soaked with water. Sika Garri was therefore a clever way of branding this money multiplier scheme.

20 See YouTube video "Call me Rev. Dr. Prophetess Evangelist Mama Pat – Agradaa changes name" (www.youtube.com/watch?v=zLpVaPE3Qx8).

As generations of chief priests have gone out at dawn to engage with new clients in the physical public sphere, so do the new priests go onto social media, the contemporary public sphere, to engage with (prospective) clients. These new practices uphold the cultural tradition of reinventing healing traditions. They change with the times by reading society and the health marketplace, which is becoming increasingly global, strategically borrowing from competitors and giving people what they want, locally and in far-flung places.

"Diabetes Last Stop"

In the early 2010s, a signpost began appearing in various locations, outside hospitals and at strategic road junctions, in Accra and Tema. It had a simple design: the words Diabetes Last Stop painted in black and red, and beneath these words an arrow and a telephone number (Figure 2.5). I first saw the signpost outside Tema General Hospital, located within a collection of signposts advertising a variety of health-related and general goods and services.

The signpost was unique in its simplicity, but it displayed a clear understanding, and creative adaptation, of local discourse around transportation and also of healing as a journey with a definitive endpoint. For the majority of Ghanaians who use public transport, 'last stop' signals the final destination for a *tro-tro* (public transport bus) or taxi route. The

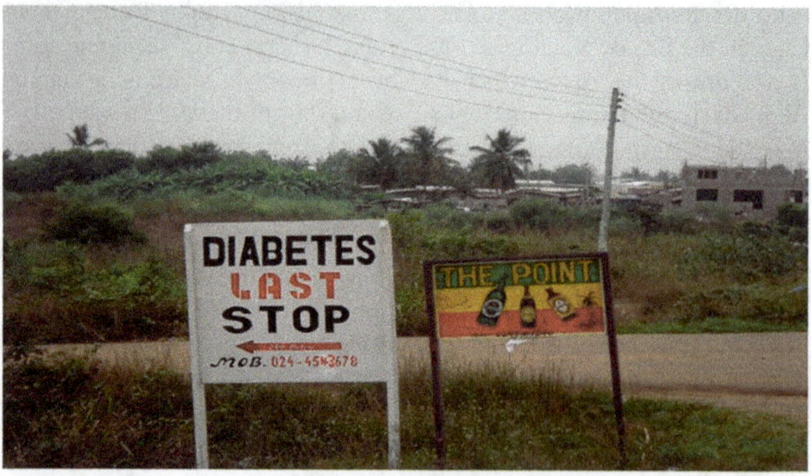

Figure 2.5 Diabetes Last Stop signpost, Tema.

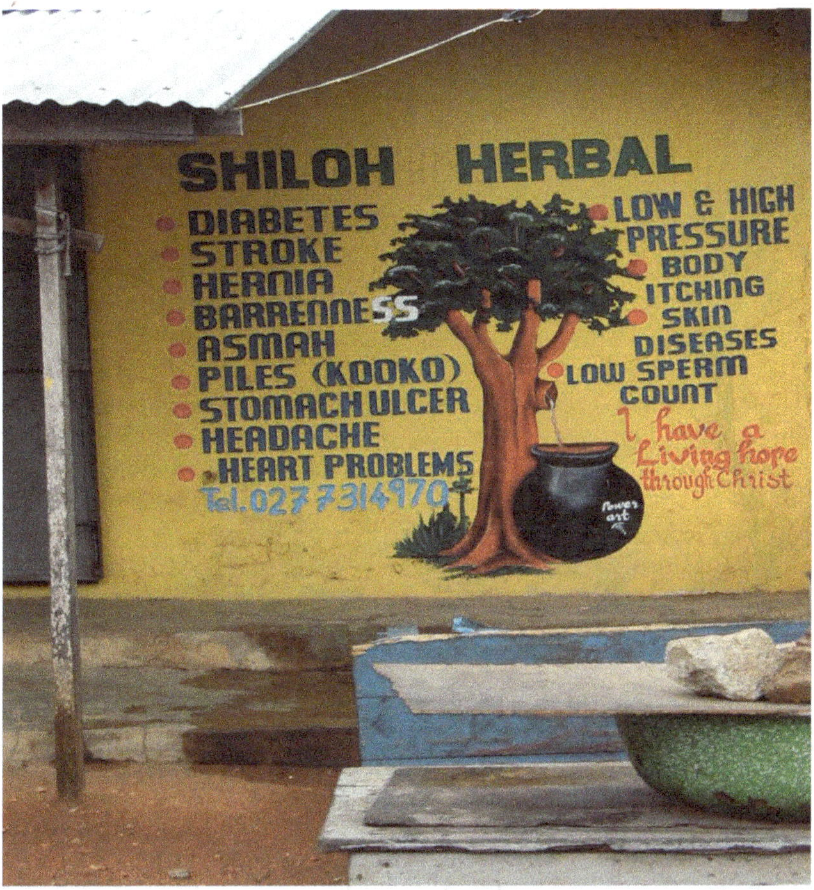
SHILOH HERBAL
DIABETES
STROKE
HERNIA
BARRENNESS
ASMAH
PILES (KOOKO)
STOMACH ULCER
HEADACHE
HEART PROBLEMS
Tel.0277314970
LOW & HIGH PRESSURE
BODY ITCHING
SKIN DISEASES
LOW SPERM COUNT
I have a Living hope through Christ
Power art

Figure 2.6 Shiloh Herbal wall advert, Kintampo.

signpost suggested that calling the telephone number would start a journey towards a cure for diabetes. It was also unique in its focus on offering a specialist service for one condition: diabetes.

The majority of signposts for herbal medicine services focus on more generalist practices. The advert for Shiloh Herbal painted on the wall of the centre located in Kintampo (Figure 2.6) is typical of this dominant set.

In *Oxford Street City Life and the Itineraries of Transnationalism* Ghanaian literary scholar Ato Quayson (2014) describes Oxford Street – an iconic commercial street in Accra – as an archive upon which "a veritable galaxy of mottoes and slogans on lorries, cars, pushcarts, and other surfaces are frequently to be encountered" (p.130). Mottoes and slogans, Quayson observes, are a

> "distinctive feature of Accra and of many African urban environments". They "extend from a domain of oral performativity and reach into the domain of writing, such that the process of reading them requires an innovative understanding of their mixed genres and the orality/literacy spectrum from which they draw their meaning(s)" (p.130).

Advertising by the herbal industry employs slogans, mottoes and signposts within the 'orality/literacy spectrum' to great effect. Signposts and billboards advertising versions of the 'Diabetes Last Stop' and Shiloh Herbal's cures for multiple conditions proliferate along major roads, at transport yards, in markets, outside hospitals, churches and mosques across the country. Fly posters appear on temporary hoardings. Leaflets are pinned on trees. Itinerant herbalists advertise on public transport and in hospital car parks, waiting rooms and corridors, employing a mix of creative methods – storytelling, comedy, singing and dance. The more sophisticated herbal centres, such as Top Herbal and Agbeve Clinic, apply a multi-pronged approach, blending radio and television adverts, newspaper adverts and signposts. Instead of deploying lone itinerant herbalists to advertise on public transport, they use branded vans with loudspeakers blaring out messages of healing. The Agbeve Tonic van (Figure 2.7) begins its drive through low-income neighbourhoods in Accra like Ga Mashie, Labadi and Osu at 6 a.m. Products are advertised on the van – the classic Agbeve Tonic, Agbeve Capsules, Agbeve Balm and Agbeve Herbal Tea. A pre-recorded advert is played loudly on speakers fixed to the van. In the advert, a woman speaking Ga and Twi details how Agbeve Tonic can cure a collection of health conditions, including kwashiorkor (a childhood disease of micronutrient deficiency), diabetes and migraines (Figure 2.8).

When I conducted my doctoral fieldwork in Nkoranza in 2001, I was granted permission to observe one popular herbal clinic, where queues formed early in the morning and built up throughout the day. In the consulting room, the herbalist sat behind a desk in a white laboratory coat with a stethoscope around his neck. A microscope sat on the desk. He had no training in laboratory sciences. Both instruments were used in performative ways – like Ataa's use of the mirror, *wokui* and cowrie shells – a gentle tug of the stethoscope as he asked questions, a vague wave towards the microscope to emphasise the scientific basis of his diagnostic expertise. During his breaks, the herbalist walked around the town centre in his white laboratory coat and answered to calls of 'doctor'.

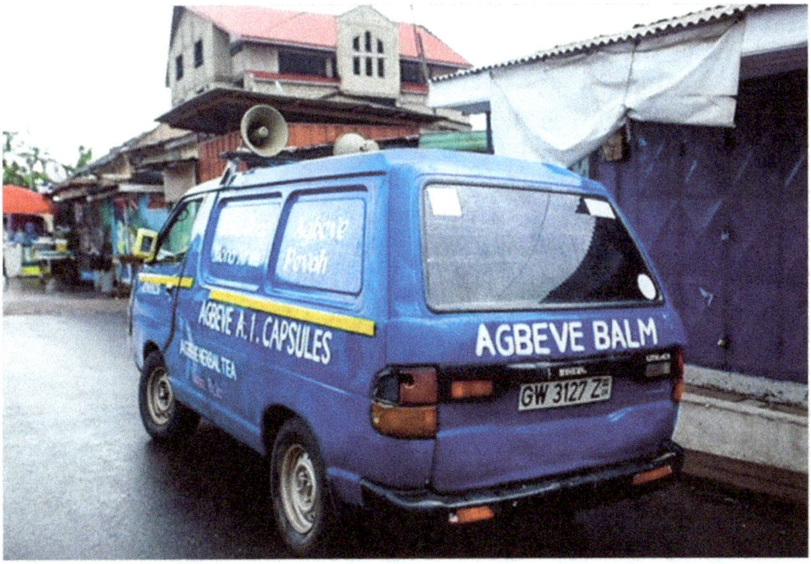

Figure 2.7 Agbeve Tonic van, Osu, Accra.

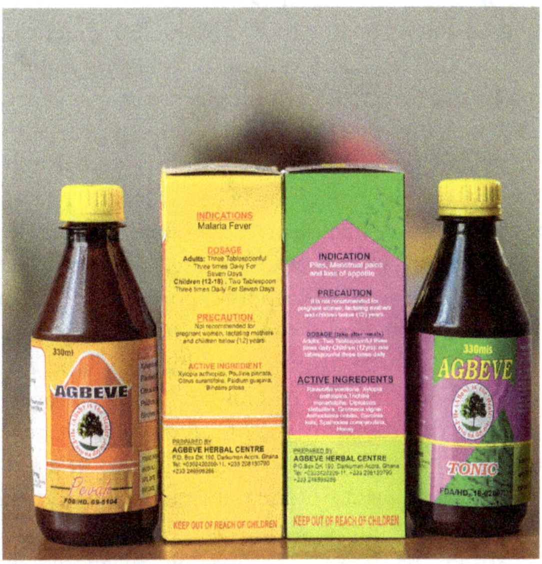

Figure 2.8 Agbeve Tonics approved by the Food and Drugs Authority (FDA). These two products treat 'malaria fever' and 'piles, menstrual pains and loss of appetite'. The mobile adverts promote Agbeve Tonic as "an ancient remedy that treats all ailments and diseases", and an extended range of conditions: high blood pressure, diabetes, rheumatism and poor vision (See Appendix 3c for the full transcript of the advert).

At the time, herbal clinics like the one in Nkoranza were few in number. Now, the number of herbal clinics in Ghana is in the thousands. Crude and processed herbal medicines that are mass-produced for domestic use and export constitute a multi-million-dollar global industry (van Andel et al., 2012). The big clinics employ multidisciplinary teams, including graduates from the recently established herbal medicine bachelor's degree programme at the Kwame Nkrumah University of Science and Technology (KNUST). Mass-produced herbal medicines are submitted for official testing, approval and certification at the Food and Drugs Authority (FDA) based in Accra, and the Centre for Plant Medicine Research (CPMR) based in Mampong-Akwapim in the Eastern Region. Some herbalists undergo training in complementary therapies from Asian countries. Some buy fake doctorates from a grey market of fake doctorate-conferring institutions and receive honorary doctorates from the international honorary doctorate production mill. Some complete courses in Christian theology and take on public identities as Charismatic Christian apostles, prophets or pastors, in order to provide faith-based herbal treatment services. Hyphenated identities such as herbalist-prophets and herbalist-apostles have become commonplace.

American anthropologist Damien Droney (2022) described two herbal clinics he observed in Accra in 2013. These clinics were run by Chief Executive Officers (CEOs). Each clinic was 'religiously affiliated', one to an evangelical Christian church, the other to a mosque. One was a single-site clinic that sold imported medicines and specialised in infertility treatment. The CEO had been trained by his herbalist father in the Ashanti Region and studied herbal medicine in Japan. The other was part of a chain of clinics, mass-manufactured its own herbal medicines and specialised in post-stroke rehabilitation. Here, the CEO, named Victor, who "had made his fortune in import-export, insurance and lumber" (p.235) before entering the herbal medicine industry, introduced Droney to a new diagnostic machine manufactured by the Chinese company GR Hunter called the Metatron. The machine, a recent innovation in global alternative medicine developed by a Russian scientist – and also called a non-linear diagnostic system (NLS) – operated by 'sensing electromagnetic frequencies' that could detect "hidden infirmities in the human body" (p.235). During a trial diagnosis with a patient, a reverend minister who had a history of stroke and diabetes, the machine diagnosed 'prostatitis and a respiratory infection'. The machine was switched to treatment mode after the CEO declared to all present that "The machine can treat conditions as well!"

> An image of the reverend's blood cells came on screen, with some highlighted problem areas. Soon, a hunting target floated across the highlighted areas, and the screen flashed. The reverend repeatedly exclaimed, 'Jesus Christ!', while others in the room expressed their astonishment. Victor began speaking of the cost of the machine, asserting that it was actually cheap given the amazing results that it provided. Finally, when the machine reported that the patient was 42% healed, Victor said, 'This is magic! It's magic!' (p.236).

There is a clear creative path linking the "performance of technological spectacle" (Droney, 2022, p.235) with big, expensive equipment like the Metatron, the use of smaller 'non-spectacular technologies' like the stethoscopes and microscopes in a Nkoranza clinic ten years prior, and Ataa's performance with *wokui* in Labadi in the 1980s.[21] In all of these encounters, the performance is integral to diagnosis, treatment and promised cures.

There is also constant evolution of positioning and purpose in the pluralistic healthcare system. Typically, and as we saw in Nkoranza, there is professional competition not only between indigenous healing systems and biomedicine, but also within the indigenous healing systems, particularly on conditions with perceived spiritual underpinnings. And in keeping with strategic borrowing from the culturally distant, the contemporary targets of professional competition have shifted to the global writ large. The herbal clinics Droney observed worked towards setting themselves apart from local medical systems and positioned themselves "with alternative medical practitioners around the world" (p.244), and by extension to a multi-billion-dollar global industry. Similarly, contemporary shrine priests like Kwaku Bonsam, or reformed ones like Nana Agradaa, positioned themselves within a globalising African Traditional Religion movement or new hybrid religious models.

As more Ghanaians live with chronic conditions over long periods of time and tell their complicated stories of lived experience and healer-shopping, public understanding is expanding on what works and what harms in herbal clinics, shrines and faith healing spaces. These discrepancies have become so well known in Ghanaian society that "fake pastor" and "fake herbalist" have become recurring tropes in popular culture (Meyer, 2015; Shipley, 2009). Films and television dramas feature themes of thwarted healing journeys for

[21] Droney describes the modernisation of Ayurveda, drawing on Projit Mukarji's historical account: "small non-spectacular technologies like watches, thermometers and microscopes became material artefacts around which a 'braiding' of knowledges occurred, producing modern Ayurveda out of the conjuncture of historically contingent social structures and situated actors" (p.234).

protagonists.[22] These stories are often presented as satire or cautionary tales. A recent comedy sketch titled "How Ghana Herbal Hospitals Advertise Themselves on TV" was posted on Twitter (now X) in August 2022 by the Ghanaian comedian and social media influencer Mempeasem President. The sketch, performed in Twi, satirised all the elements of previous examples of creative innovation within the herbal medicine industry (excerpt in Box 2.1). This sketch laid bare the problematic aspects of creativity and innovation in the herbal industry, as well as the vital functions of lay scrutiny and scepticism of healing environments.

Box 2.1 How Ghana Herbal Hospitals Advertise Themselves on TV – excerpt of a comedy sketch.

Me ma mo akwaaba eba Kpomegbe Herbal Centre. Y'asoeyɛ ha deɛ, sɛ yareɛ bia eha wo bia no, wode ba ha nkoa dea, yebe tu aseɛ ama wokoraa.	I welcome you all to Kpomegbe Herbal Center. Here, no matter the sickness, once you come to us, we cure it for you.
Obi wɔ hɔ a, ose dokta me ti na ɛyɛ me ya. Nanso ɔba ha na ye de no fa mfideɛ no mu a, ye tumi hu yareɛ ahodoɔ nso a, ɛsan ɛha no paa.	Someone might say, doctor, I have a headache but when he comes here and we scan him with our machines, we are able to diagnose other sicknesses he may be suffering from.
Yɛwɔ adokter akukudam a ɔmo akɔ suapɔn mu ako sua adeɛ ama ɔmo nimdeɛ ɛko akyi.	We have competent doctors who are highly trained.
Yareɛ ben? Sɛ barima a wadwodwo, mogya boroso, sisi yadeɛ, honam ani nyarewa ne kooko ɛne asikyere yare3. Na netitriw paa, yareɛ paa yetatu aseɛ paa, ene ɛtwo. HIV deɛ Kpomegbe Herbal Center yentumi ɛnsa saa yareɛ no bi but yebetumi asoso ano ama wo nkakra nkakra. Eno sei, wo de sai obi kora mpo no aa. nhyɛda ɛnyɛ serios saa.	What is the sickness? Low sperm count, hypertension, waist problems, skin diseases, piles, diabetes and especially hernia. For HIV, Kpomegbe Herbal Center can't cure it but we can give you medications to control it. With that, even when you infect someone, it won't be that serious.

[22] See, for example, renowned Ghanaian director Kwaw Ansah's 2013 film *Praising The Lord Plus One* – or its trailer on YouTube (www.youtube.com/watch?v=OXOzSovK3nE). At the end of gospel singer Joyce Blessing's video for her song *Repent*, she acts in a short skit as a false prophet who pays a team of women to pose as recipients of healing during church services (see www.youtube .com/watch?v=CHCevrhEm5A).

Ebi nso aa spiritual marriage. Yɛ wo neɛma bi nso a yebetumi de asa spiritual marriage. Yɛ wɔ condom a woda aa wo betumi de ahye sɛnea ɛbɛyɛ a maame water bi anaa sunsum bi ne wo bɛda a wonya ebia nsusuanso bone bia a ɛha woabrabɔ.	For spiritual marriages, we have what it takes to cure that. We have condoms that when worn at night, marine spirits and other evil spirits won't have any bad effects on your life after having sex with you.
Y'agye abodin nkrataa ɛna yɛsan nso wɔ abosobɔdeɛ a yɛkɔgyee no wo China man mu a y'asan agye bi nso ɛwo US ɛne UK a ɛkyerɛsɛ yen nnwuma a yedi no, ɛso ani bebre ɛwɔ wiase afanan nyinaa.	We have acquired certifications. We also have awards from China, US and UK which proves that our work has been recognised globally.
Wo ba na wobusa akolaa kora sɛ wo ko Kpomegbe Herbal Centre a, omo bɛkyerɛ wo. Afei nso wobetumi afrɛ yen wɔ 0204985 3721.	When you ask even a child, about Kpomegbe Herbal Center, you will be directed to our centre. You can also call us on 0204985 3721.
Kpomegbe Herbal Centre anaa, yɛ yɛ bue!	Kpomegbe Herbal Centre, we are great!
	Source: @AsieduMends. Twitter (now X) account of Mempeasem President, Comic Act/Social Media Influencer.

Selling Sickness Meets Re-inventions of Healing Traditions

The German anthropologist Birgit Meyer (2015), who has conducted extensive ethnographic work on Ewe healing systems as well as Pentecostal Christian movements in Ghana, defines imaginaries as:

> interlaced sets of collective representations around particular issues – such as the nation, ethnicity, the city, the family, sickness and wellbeing, the divine, the occult, and so on – that underpin the moral and intellectual schemes and sensory modes that govern people's way of being in the world and that thereby "make" this world (p.14).

Imaginaries, she further notes, "are woven around diverse cultural forms such as objects, texts, pictures, words, songs, smells – in principle anything that exists in the world and is an object of perception and sensation" (p.15) and of "emotions and semantics" (p.19).

In the Akan and Ga communities featured in this chapter, spirits and supernatural beings are objects of perception, sensation, emotions and semantics (Akyeampong, 1995; Meyer, 2015; Mullings, 1984). Much of the creative work indigenous healers do converges with the workings of spirits and realms of the supernatural: entities and spaces that are unseen and invisible but felt, feared, talked about and battled with. I define spiritual imaginaries as representations of spiritual and supernatural phenomena that shape health beliefs, healing journeys, healing encounters and healing environments. If we apply the concept of cognitive polyphasia to this representational space, then spiritual imaginaries constitute a form of knowledge. Spiritual imaginaries can stand alone as a concrete knowledge modality (like science, politics or common sense) or weave together elements within a range of knowledge systems. For example, in healing environments, the spiritual phenomena that healers and clients perceive, sense, feel and speak of connect the "symbolic and physiological", "sacred and mundane", "visible and invisible" (Mullings, 1984) aspects of healing. In these instances, spiritual imaginaries straddle, to draw on Goody's (1975, 1987) formulation, basic, traditional and transformational knowledge.

'Selling sickness' meets 'reinventions of healing traditions' in these symbolic and material spaces. Healers sell healing for a variety of ailments and especially those of ambiguous provenance that biomedicine cannot cure. Healers strive to make the unknown known, the invisible visible, the unfamiliar familiar, whether these are newly encountered or already known outside or within social and physical boundaries. And they do this by all means at their disposal, but often with the tools of creative imagination and expression. The reinvention of healing traditions is a creative process: it requires the gathering and interpretation of social facts, borrowing strategically from rival systems and thinking, imagining, conceptualising, planning and marketing. Healers advertise their superior healing skills – on the streets, at festivals, on traditional and social media, and in private consulting spaces. Storytelling, singing, visual art, sculpture, bodily art, the use of costume and of bodily performance serve important functions in these strategies.

Artists also play a pivotal role in the social construction of healing environments. In the examples presented in this chapter, we see the work of sculptors, costumers, sign painters, musicians, singers and advertisement copywriters. Some come from long family lines of master artists who work in the space of sacred arts – those who carve out representations of the gods, sew the ritual garments for priests and paint murals on shrine walls. Others are formally trained or self-taught and produce "popular arts" (Barber, 1987): the sign painters who produce the bulk of signposts for herbalists and shrine priests, contemporary musicians, singers or voice artists who provide background music or create slogans for radio, television and mobile van adverts, and comedians creating satirical sketches on social media about the limits of selling healing.

CHAPTER 3

Mr Wise and Mr Foolish Go to Town

"Ɔhɔho ani akɛseakɛse, nanso onhuu hwee.

The stranger's eyes are very big with looking, but she/he doesn't see anything.

Akan Proverb

In June 1944, a letter arrived for the Gold Coast Governor, Sir Alan Cuthbert Maxwell Burns, from the Colonial Office at Downing Street, London. The letter, written by Mr Noel Sabine, proposed to dispatch a silent 35 mm film on the subject of "venereal disease amongst Africans".[1] The film had been originally produced in South Africa on syphilis prevention for mining communities and had been titled *The Two Brothers*. For the West African colonies the original title was changed, for unexplained reasons, to *Mr Wise and Mr Foolish Go to Town*. The story was simple, as the letter outlined:

> The film attempts to point out the moral of two Africans – Mr Wise and Mr Foolish – who both contract the disease – syphilis – but who separately go about their cures in different ways with fortunate and unfortunate consequences respectively to themselves and their families.

Two further facts emerged in subsequent communication. Both men had contracted syphilis from their extra-marital affairs. Mr Wise went to see a colonial doctor and was cured; Mr Foolish went to see a "medicine man" (i.e. a shrine priest or herbalist) and remained sick.

In order for the adaption to be approved, several letters were written to the heads of the important institutions of the day: Acting Director of Medical Services, the Director of Education, Director of the Chamber of Mines, and leaders of the Missions and military. A Special Board, made up of a subset of the letter recipients, was established to assess the suitability of

[1] Public Records and Archives Administration Department (PRAAD) CSO 11/3129.

the film for local audiences. Eventually a viewing was held at the Rex Cinema in Accra for a broad group of elite adult men: "Missionaries, lawyers, businessmen, press representatives, African inspectors of schools and teachers."[2] The reaction to the letters and the viewing was mixed.

The Acting Director of Medical Services, argued that gonorrhoea was a much bigger public health problem than syphilis[3]:

> Gonorrhoea would be a much better venereal disease to caution people against than "syphilis" (*quotation marks in original*). Syphilis is still comparatively uncommon, but its incidence is, apparently, increasing. Gonorrhoea is however known to all; its incidence is widespread and its effects a menace of the first order.

He also observed that the uniform worn by Mr Wise's girlfriend was too similar to the uniforms worn by Gold Coast nurses.

> it is a pity that "Mr Wise's" lady love appeared in uniform indistinguishable from that of an African nurse in the medical department. This point will doubtless strike everybody

Both he and other viewers suggested the filmmakers change the character of the girlfriend to a 'housemaid' wearing different clothing to avoid the wrath of Gold Coast nurses who, they appeared to suggest, would not take kindly to being depicted as girlfriends of married men.

Others felt that if the narration was too serious, the film might make people laugh too much, which would defeat its educational purpose. Indeed, there had been some "sniggering" (said Mr John Wilson, Gold Coast PRO) at the viewing. For those who were of the view that Gold Coasters were "too primitive" the voice-over needed to be 'done by an educated person with an authoritative voice'. Some suggestions were made on suitable audiences for the film: 'miners in Tarkwa' (a gold mining town) "schools and colleges, youth societies and the like."[4]

Ultimately, the consensus from local experts was that not only were both men foolish, the film itself was also foolish.

MR JOHN WILSON: "the film shows both Mr Wise and Mr Foolish making their arrangements for... illicit relationships, without a hint that they are acting foolishly."

DIRECTOR OF EDUCATION: "it seems strange that no section dealing with the prevention of disease was included in the film...If ever special films are prepared for West Africa, I feel it would be most wise to include such a section."

[2] PRAAD CSO 11/3129. [3] PRAAD CSO 11/3129. [4] PRAAD CSO 11/3129.

On behalf of the governor, Mr Wilson wrote very detailed recommendations to Mr Sabine on how to change the film's content, language and delivery. It is difficult to know whether miners in Tarkwa, school children or youth societies ever saw the film – there is no further material on the campaign in the archival records after Mr Wilson's final letter in October 1944. But the months-long discussions and anxiety around having the film backfire spectacularly across all social classes in the Gold Coast suggests that the original idea had not been thought through critically. And once some thought had been applied to content, context and impact, the Downing Street officials and their allies decided, quite wisely, to quit while they were ahead.

Mr Wise and Mr Foolish Go to Town is one of the more prominent colonial attempts to apply arts to public health communication. It stands out as a case study because the records clearly track the way the colonial public health – and public policy – machinery operated, from conceptualisation of ideas to implementation of a project. The letters and reports highlighted the racialised, gendered and class dimensions of colonial policy making. They also revealed the ideological tensions between colonial medicine and indigenous medicine.

In the archives, and in social history accounts on colonial era health interventions, other arts-based projects are documented. Some were implemented prior to *Mr Wise and Mr Foolish*, others after. American social historian Jean Allman (1994) describes a Baby Show launched in Kumasi in 1925, by the Senior Sanitary Officer, Dr Selwyn-Clarke. The show, which ran annually and by 1929 had 'transformed completely into a mechanism of social regulation, if not social control, of colonial motherhood' (p.29) was part of a broader "British imperialist project of making 'proper mothers' at home and in the colonies" (p.25). This 'mothercraft' project, was entrusted with and implemented by 'maternal imperialists'. These were 'missionaries, nurses, teachers and women medical officers' who conducted baby bathing demonstrations, as well as cookery (with a focus on British pancakes and biscuits), sewing, gardening and reading lessons in colonial mission spaces as well as in the private homes of Asante mothers.

In the 1940s and 1950s, food fairs were organised in Accra and other towns, at which local and regional cuisines were displayed and sampled. Some cuisines were collated for the publication of a colonial cookbook titled Gold Coast Nutrition and Cookery (Gold Coast Government, 1953)).[5]

[5] Although Gold Coast Nutrition and Cookery featured Gold Coast, African, European and Caribbean recipes, the cover showed an aproned young girl making pastry, possibly building on

There were letters related to themed art competitions for children (to aid child development) and the promotion of health and sanitation via newspaper cartoons and adverts (Figure 3.1).

In many cases on record, ideas were developed in London usually at the Colonial Office at Downing Street or at a public relations firm in central London – with some minor contributions by West African subsidiaries – and brought to the Gold Coast for tweaking. What tied these arts-based interventions together, though, was their embeddedness in the broader colonial medicine project. This project was not benign.

Franz Fanon, the Algerian psychiatrist, revolutionary and post-colonial theorist, theorized about the way African psychological realities were conditioned by relations of racialized power and violence during the colonial era. He called these intersections of psychological and socio-political conditions 'the psychic life of the colonial encounter' (Fanon, 1963). This psychic life was double-edged.

From the European side, colonial medicine was often violent. The story on sleeping sickness in countries colonized by the French is particularly instructive. Painful examinations, such as spinal taps, were performed on entire villages often under gun point by the soldiers protecting travelling medical teams. Treatments, such as the drugs Atoxyl and Lomidine, were more harmful than the disease itself, causing blindness in 20 per cent of recipients and death in many more (Lowes and Montero, 2021). In the Gold Coast, sleeping sickness campaigns introduced new infections in Northern communities (Bannister, 2021). At the heart of public health campaigns and medical experimentations and treatments was the notion of the African as 'a pathological museum'. American historian Melissa Graboyes (2015, p.xii), observes that this notion captured the European researcher's amazement at

> the collection of germs, pathogens, viruses, parasites, and other abnormal and unusual diseases likely to be found in a single African body

Biological specimens from African bodies – bodily fluids, diseased organs, skeletons and so on – were transported to actual 'pathology museums' in European medical schools, in Britain, France, Belgium and elsewhere. There, trainee doctors and medical researchers who planned to work in

the British focus of cookery projects run by British women missionaries in Asante and elsewhere, as described by Allman (1994). The production of cookbooks was an experiment that was deployed across the British colonies in Africa and India to engineer 'national cuisines' (McCann, 2010).

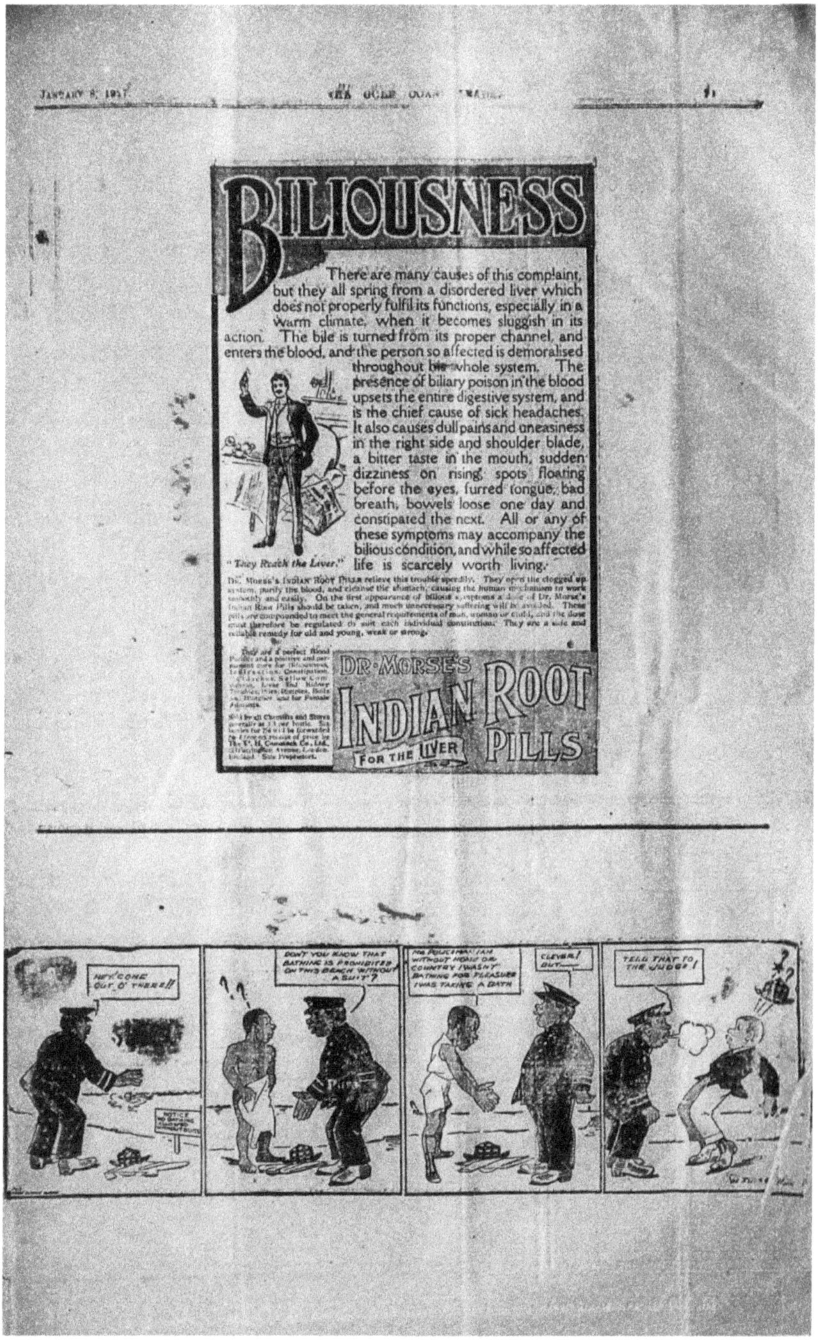

Figure 3.1 'No bathing allowed without suits' Cartoon, *Gold Coast Leader*, 8 January 1927.

the tropics were able to see representations of diseases they were unlikely to see and could barely imagine in their own countries.

What colonial medicine did to Africa was one side of a complex story. The other side is how African communities anticipated, saw through, worked around and resisted medical violence, in very similar ways to political resistance to colonialism itself. Veteran Ghanaian journalist Cameron Duodu recalls his childhood days in colonial Gold Coast, when "all the 'smart' people in our villages tended to run away from vaccination" because colonial health authorities were "uncommunicative" and "behaved like gods" (Duodu, 2004).

When arts-based health interventions were implemented in cities and villages in the Gold Coast, Asante and Northern Territories, they carried the same air of 'uncommunicative' 'god-like' behaviour; and they were seen by local communities as an extension of the colonial medical project. Projects that sought to impose a British way of doing things were rejected, or were transformed into versions that served local needs. Allman (1994) writes that Asante mothers negotiated their encounters with maternal imperialists on their own terms. In a 1942 report, J.B. Kirk,[6] Director of Gold Coast Medical Services, noted that in Europe,

> the weighing centre is generally the place where demonstrations in the care and management of infants are conducted, cookery lessons given, dress-making classes organised and the general welfare of children impressed upon all who attend there for these purposes (Allman, 1994, p.33).

In Kumasi, Asante mothers had entirely different ideas about the functions of weighing centres. They,

> exhibited profound disinterest in the mothercraft agenda with which the Kumasi Centre began operations. They were not ambivalent, however, concerning their access to medical care alternatives. Using the pressure of their numbers at the health care clinics and the absence of their numbers at weighing clinics and mothercraft lectures, they fundamentally transformed the agenda of the Centre (Allman, 1994, p.33).

Today, the major arts-based health interventions in Ghana are embedded in the broader global health project, and are funded by global health institutions.[7] These projects are conceptualised in similar ways to their colonial predecessors.

[6] PRAAD CSO 11/7/28.

[7] See Appendix 1 for the results of a scoping review of arts and health studies in Ghana.

Arts and the Psychopolitics of Global Health Encounters

A team of American and Ghanaian public health researchers evaluated the impact of a National Handwashing Campaign, also branded National Truly Clean Hands Campaign, which aimed to 'market hygiene behaviours' to Ghanaian women (Scott et al., 2008). The campaign was a multi-site intervention, led by the London School of Hygiene and Tropical Medicine (LSHTM), which applied a standardised multi-media approach to improving handwashing in seven countries in Africa, Asia and Latin America: Ghana, Senegal, Tanzania, Nepal, Vietnam, Columbia and Peru. The conceptual framework blended ideas in marketing and behavioural science. A news release on the LSHTM website stated that the project "was abandoning the traditional 'health education' approach, which [had] been tried, without success in the past, in favour of a commercial, marketing-led approach."[8] This new approach was a "Global Public-Private Partnership for Handwashing" between "LSHTM, UNICEF, the World Bank, national and local government partners in Ghana and international and national soap companies including Unilever, PZ Cussons and Getrade".

In Ghana, the campaign was implemented in all the ten regions in December 2003. Following the dominant methodology of multi-national arts-based public health projects, the project had two elements. A national level mass media campaign involved television adverts in Twi and English, radio adverts in "10 local languages" (p.394) and billboards. Community engagement in five regions, was conducted in partnership with the Community Water and Sanitation Agency (GCWSA), and involved "direct consumer contact (DCC) events", posters and stickers distributed at events, schools and through GCWSA "extension services" and "launch activities across all regions and 120 of 138 districts" (p.394). The research team collaborated with a local advertising agency, Lintas Ghana, to develop mass media campaign tools. The campaign song, called *Hohorowonsa* (Wash your hands, in Twi), was played on radio and television adverts and during community engagement events.

Hohoro wonsa, fa samina yɛ,	Wash your hand, use soap,
hohoro wonsa, fa samina ka,	wash your hands, use soap,
hohoro wonsa ooo	wash your hands,

[8] Campaigners abandon health education for marketing in drive to promote lifesaving properties of soap | LSHTM (last accessed 29th August 2023).

hohoro wonsa ooo	wash your hands,
Fa samena yɛ, saa na ɛyɛ	Use soap, that is right

(Excerpt of the song)[9]

The evaluation was conducted with 497 mothers of children aged under five, in the five study communities where community engagement events had been convened: Greater Accra, Ashanti, Western, Volta and Upper East regions. A structured questionnaire co-designed with GCWSA and Business Interactive Ghana, a market research agency, covered issues of "reach, message recall, interpretation and reported behaviour" (p.394). Focus groups and in-depth interview, conducted with a subset of the survey respondents, examined "likes and dislikes relating to campaign components and reported behaviour change" (p.394). The general finding was that the campaign was accepted, the arts-based methods played a major role (the song in particular was remembered by all), and there was evidence of behaviour modification. Some results were statistically significant.

In the general discussion, the authors observed the following:

> Prior to our campaign, *handwashing was largely a social norm, but the inclusion of soap in the ritual was not.* Many respondents reported that they were left deeply impressed by the campaign content, *previously believing that water alone was enough to clean hands after visiting the toilet and before eating. Having not known the importance of soap*, many said that they felt uncomfortable when exposed to the campaign materials which now make them realise that they must use soap (p.400, emphasis added).

The statement that 'many respondents' did not 'know the importance of soap' was presented as incontrovertible fact. The only reference provided to this statement was an unpublished report of the Campaign's formative research. The statement also contradicted the LSHTM news release which stated that Ghanaians were "major consumers of soap". Indeed, in the target study communities, there are long standing traditions and rituals on bodily and environmental cleanliness that involve water and soap. The local production of soaps like '*Alata Samina*' (or Black Soap), for example, has a long history. Today, these local soaps are not only used and sold locally, they are also sold to a growing international market of diaspora Africans and the soap-making process has joined a growing list of tourist activities that promote culture-immersion.[10] The authors did not engage

[9] (617) Ghana Handwashing Promotion Advertisement – YouTube.

[10] Global Mamas, an international NGO that operates in Ghana and other African countries produces and sells their version of Black Soap, called Dandy Lion Black Soap using methods perfected by

with these local systems of knowledge and practices around bodily and environmental cleanliness. They did not mention water poverty or other structural factors that may have influenced changing behaviours around bodily and environmental cleanliness within the cohort of study evaluation participants. Their interpretation of the study findings was disconnected from the cultures and histories of the study communities. The sub-text of the study – generating revenue for international and national soap companies through a Global Public-Private Partnership for Handwashing – was absent in the paper.

Ghanaian communications scholar Kwasi Ansu-Kyeremeh and colleagues (2016), citing Brazilian educationist Paulo Freire, refer to research practices displayed in projects like the Truly Clean Hands Campaign as the "banking education" method of health communication:

> Messages seem basically instructional and prescriptive; demanding of recipients to act and not, for example, find out, analyse, think or make suggestions about things. Intended receivers [are] not challenged to positively exploit their experiences. It is the typical encyclopaedic or Freire "banking education" approach to communication which assumes a know all message source and a know-nothing message destination (p.7).

Even when local (Ghanaian) research collaborators and artists are engaged, as they were with Truly Clean Hands, the perception of their proximity to a 'know-nothing message destination' restricts the scope of their conceptual and practical contributions. Across the African continent, arts-based global health interventions – for HIV/AIDS, malaria, reproductive health and other major health conditions – employ the same conceptual and interpretive approaches (Bunn et al., 2020). Even those that espouse 'participatory' principles and draw on local arts traditions employ an instrumental approach, where "participants have no authority to decide on their own priorities but remain exposed to participation as a form of subjection, if not tyranny" (Chinyowa, 2015, p.18). Typically these projects lead communities "into participating in workshops using 'folk' songs, dances, poems and stories that have already been planned for them" (Abdulla, 2016, p.459). Artists commissioned to develop messaging for such projects often "become concerned with creating a final product that will satisfy funding agencies, neglecting the creative process and in-depth engagement with the social problem to be addressed" (Boneh and Jaganath, 2011, p.456). Kennedy Chinyowa (2015), citing Robert

soap makers in Suhum, a town in the Eastern Region (see https://globalmamas.org/handcrafting/african-black-soap).

Chambers (1997), contrasts instrumental participation with transformational participation: "the instrumental paradigm means that 'they' (local people) participate in 'our' project as opposed to the transformational paradigm in which 'we' participate in 'their' project."

The banking education approach, as Paulo Freire (1970/2017) noted in the *Pedagogy of the Oppressed*, is 'anti-dialogical':

> For the anti-dialogical banking educator, the question of content simply concerns the program about which he will discourse to his students, and he answers his own question, by organizing his own program (p.66).

Education that leads to social transformation requires a dialogical approach:

> For the dialogical problem-posing teacher-student, the program content of education is neither gift nor an imposition – bits of information to be deposited in the students – but rather the organized, systematized and developed "re-presentation" to individuals of the things about which they want to know more (p.66).

Freire argues that dialogue has to be driven, on both sides of the encounter, by "love", "humility" and "faith" (pp.62–63). The dialoguers must engage in critical thinking that recognises the "concrete, existential, present situation of real people" (p.66). The encounter has to engender trust (p.64).

This chapter was prefaced with the Akan proverb that speaks to the distorted gaze of an outsider: "Ɔhɔho ani akɛseakɛse, nanso onhuu hwee/ the stranger's eyes are very big with looking, but s/he doesn't see anything". The proverb delineates an Akan social psychology of insider-outside encounters. 'Seeing' has a double meaning: it refers to sight *and* understanding. The stranger's way of seeing is understood by the host. But the host's way of being is unlikely to be understood – and by extension transformed – by the stranger who looks but sees nothing. The Freirean elements of dialogical engagement, from both sides of the encounter, are implicit in the proverb.

In Global Health, there is a particular way of looking at and not quite seeing African communities in full colour, texture and flow. This distorted gaze – illustrated clearly by the Truly Clean Hands campaign in Ghana and other continental examples – dates back to the colonial era.

Colonial medicine established a trope of 'Africa as a conduit for infection'. Notions such as the African as a "walking pathological museum" have morphed into contemporary versions, such as the 'African AIDS epidemic' (Barz and Cohen, 2011) and more recently, 'the African COVID paradox' (see Chapter 8). For researchers developing decolonial concepts and methods in global health, this central trope maintains Africa as an enduring 'familiar alien threat' in the global imagination and informs knowledge production on Africa in global health and associated disciplines, as well as concrete political and financial choices in global governance (Greenhalgh and de-Graft Aikins, 2023; Mogaka et al., 2021).

So we may speak of "the psychic life of the contemporary global health encounter": the intersection of psychological and political dynamics mediating contemporary encounters between global health actors and local communities, as well as local experts who (claim to) represent, or advocate for, local communities. And we may also speak of two sides to the global health encounter. In the same way that Akan villagers run away from vaccination teams, or Asante women reconfigured colonial maternal and child services for their own needs, the post-colonial decades have seen several forms of resistance to global health interventions that are perceived to be harmful – from polio vaccines in Nigeria (Jegede, 2007), Ebola vaccine development in Ghana (Kummervold et al., 2017) and tetanus campaigns in Cameroon (Feldman-Savelsberg et al., 2000), to blood draws and associated biobanking procedures across the continent (Grietens et al., 2014). The psycho-political strategies employed by local communities are steeped in collective and social memory, and ignited – often during moments of personal, community and national crises – through traditions of song-making, storytelling, dance and other creative practices of the imagination.

CHAPTER 4

All Die (No) Be Die

All die be die

(A pidgin English slogan, meaning there is no distinction between a good death and a bad death)

The drama series *Things We Do for Love*, aired on Thursday nights on Ghana Television (GTV) in 2003. Written by screenwriter Edward Seddoh Jnr and directed by advertising executive Ivan Quashigah,the drama ran over 43 episodes in 30 minute segments. *Things We Do for Love* (hereafter *TWDFL*) was the first locally produced hit drama dedicated to young Ghanaians, aged sixteen and above, a demographic that was disproportionately affected by sexual and reproductive health problems, including HIV/AIDS.

The drama centred on a group of young people living in a neighbourhood in Accra. Marcia aged seventeen and her older brother Max came from a middle class family, with a doctor mother and businessman father. Dede, a mixed-race girl aged fifteen lived with her single working class mother who worked in a chop bar. Pusher and BB were older "street boys/'area boys" who orchestrated fun but morally dubious escapades in the neighbourhood. Shaker, a mixed race boy, had a hotel-owning family and drove around town in an SUV in search of 'pretty girls in Accra'. Enyonam and her brother Wisdom (who hang out with the street boys) lived, and locked horns, with a strict and emotionally abusive father. Through their relationships as siblings, friends, adversaries and romantic partners, *TWDFL* placed sexual health, including HIV/AIDS risk, within the context of important themes of the day for young people in Ghana: sexuality, sexual violence, reproductive health rights, morality, gender roles, intergenerational conflict, and beauty standards, including colourism and light-skin privilege.

The title of the show and its theme tune was inspired by the R&B song, *Things We Do for Love*, written and performed by African-American singer Horace Brown. Released in 1996, the song was a popular staple in Ghanaian nightclubs. This attention to pop culture details – and in particular the impact of African-American pop cultural trends on the local scene – informed dramatic and aesthetic choices throughout the series, including music played in their nightclubs (Hip Hop, RnB), television programmes they watched (Oprah) and magazines they read (*Essence*).

Twenty years after the last episode aired, the drama has a thriving afterlife on YouTube. To date, hundreds of thousands of people have watched cumulative episodes online. The audiences are active and engaged – they comment on storylines and their contemporary relevance. Those who were teenagers when the series aired, now in their thirties, reminisce on how the series performed the sex education role that their parents and schools did not, or could not, perform. Its social impact is similar to *Shuga*, a youth-based serial television drama that was developed over eight seasons (2009–2020) in Kenya, Nigeria, South Africa and Cote d'Ivoire reaching millions of viewers beyond these four countries (Booker et al., 2016). *TWDFL* was also a career launchpad for the young actors. Some, like Adjetey Anang who played Pusher, Majid Michel who played Shaker, and Jackie Appiah who played Enyonam, have gone on to forge major award winning careers in the Ghanaian, Nigerian and wider African film industries.

TWDFL was part of a multipronged response to the first two decades of the HIV/AIDS pandemic in Ghana by Ghana's Ministry of Health (MOH) in collaboration with donor partners, international NGOs, foreign universities and various local institutions and partners. It was conceptualised in the 'edu-tainment' genre – "the process of purposely designing and implementing a media message to both entertain and educate, in order to increase knowledge about an issue, create favourable attitudes and change overt behaviour" (Alviso, 2011, p.57). At the end of every episode there was a 'Filla' – pidgin English for 'a scoop' or gossip – segment. The segment posed a question or a set of questions that encouraged viewers to consider topical issues related to the themes in focus. This strategy layered an educational component onto the entertainment.

The first two cases of HIV infections were confirmed in March 1986 at the Noguchi Memorial Institute for Medical Research (NMIMR), a semi-autonomous institute of the University of Ghana.[1] By the time the drama aired in 2003, the national prevalence rate of HIV was 3.1 per cent (Agyei-Mensah, 2001; Boulay et al., 2008). The prevalence rate never rose above 3.1 per cent during the preceding decades; and has remained under 3 per cent in the decades that have followed. HIV is now referred to as a mixed mature

[1] NMIMR has been a national leader in clinical research since its establishment in 1979 – the institute leads infectious disease surveillance and investigations of infectious disease outbreaks including suspected cases of Ebola in 2014, and more recently of COVID-19 cases.

pandemic in Ghana. But then and now, these statistics disaggregated differently across different demographics. Young people – the target of the drama – sex workers, and men who have sex with men were more likely to have high HIV rates. Some regions, such as the Eastern and Western regions, which saw the return of large numbers of migrant sex workers from Cote d'Ivoire – had infection and death rates that exceeded the national average. These regions also saw a rise in numbers of 'HIV orphans', and grandmother headed households – a phenomenon that was more dominant in Southern Africa (Atobrah, 2016). The negative social impact of severe illness and disease stigma was deeply entrenched in communities in these regions.

I will examine how arts were incorporated into HIV/AIDS interventions, focusing on the use of mass media campaigns to raise awareness and educate, and on 'folk media' to educate and empower communities. I discuss a study, conducted by Ghanaian ethnolinguist Kwesi Yankah (2004), that applied the narrative approach to examine local knowledge and lived experience – the findings illustrated important contrasts between community and indigenous healing system responses to HIV/AIDS and official health service responses. Against the backdrop of recent reports of a resurgence of HIV infections among young Ghanaians, I will end with reflections on what these insights yield for developing more robust arts-based HIV interventions in the future.

'Love Life, Stop AIDS': Mass Media Campaigns

TWDFL was funded through a collaborative partnership between Johns Hopkins University (JHU) and the Ghana Social Marketing Fund (GSMF). During the early decades of the HIV pandemic, GSMF was a major distributor of condoms around the country. The same partners collaborated on a flagship mass media campaign programme titled Stop AIDS Love Life (hereafter SALL). SALL applied the dominant two-pronged approach to HIV/AIDS education used across African countries – a mass media campaign complemented by a community-based education drive. The mass media campaign included a song, billboards, short video documentaries and promotional materials such as leaflets, stickers, posters and t-shirts. Visual materials were branded with a SALL logo.

The signature song to the campaign, which was also titled *Stop AIDS, Love Life*, was composed by a group of prominent Ghanaian musicians and singers who collaborated under the name Ghana All Stars.[2] Running at 6.20 minutes, the song was multi-genre and multilingual. It blended

[2] List of artists and song lyrics provided in Appendix 3.

Highlife, Hiplife, Reggae and Gospel which was sung and rapped in Twi, Ewe, Fante, Ga, Hausa, pidgin English and Jamaican Patois. The video was directed in the spare visual style of global charity music videos pioneered by the Michael Jackson-led 'We are the World' campaign in 1985 – which brought together major Soul and pop artists to campaign for African famine relief through celebrity advocacy. The artistic draw in these videos is the roll call of celebrity musicians, the song lyrics, and a memorable sing along hook.

A JHU newsletter published in 2003 reported that Ghana All Stars "contributed their time and talent *gratis* to the Stop AIDS Love Life video" (p.1).[3] The core themes of SALL (as excerpted below) were the ABCs: Abstain, Be faithful, Wear a Condom. A call and response chorus led by reggae musician Shasha Marley, underscored these themes. The song applied a 'fear appeal' approach to health communication – a common, but flawed, strategy that "get [s] behind people with a big stick (lots of threat and fear) in the hope that this will drive them in the desired direction" (Job, 1988, p.163). Lyrics such as 'it is a killer' (Shasha Marley), 'this sickness. . .called AIDS. If you do not know, it will kill you' (the Ewe rapper, Chicago) served to reinforce the deadliness of the HIV virus.

Chorus
Ghana All Stars: You can maintain one lover.
Shasha Marley: Rastafarai
Ghana All Stars: it's not on, it's not in
Shasha Marley: It is a killer (x3)
Ghana All Stars: You can wait until marriage.
Shasha Marley: Can't stop knowing
Ghana All Stars: Love life, Stop Aids.

Reggie Rockstone (Twi)

Ah ɛnye ndra yi aa na me ne Kwamena ɛte ha edi nkɔmɔ yi,	Wasn't it just yesterday that Kwamena and I were chatting?
Ende mekɔ bisaa na se aa yɛse ɔkɔ	Today, I asked about him and they said he's gone.
Question, de ben na ɛyɛ no aa mo nyinaa mo ayɛ koom?	Question, what happened to him that's got you all silent?
Answer? Yareɛ keseɛ na ne din ketekete akyeno ama wawu.	Answer, that big disease with a small name caught and killed him.

[3] Johns Hopkins Bloomberg School of Public Health (2003) Communication Impact! February 2003, No. 15.

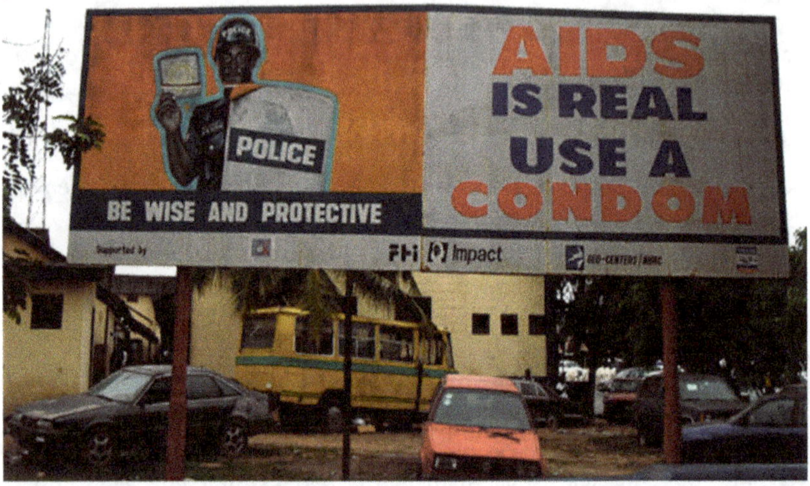
POLICE
BE WISE AND PROTECTIVE
AIDS
IS REAL
USE A
CONDOM
Impact

Figure 4.1 AIDS Is Real billboard, Sponsored by Family Health International.

SALL entered national consciousness through constant mass media play, on television and radio. The song's message was reinforced by other multi-media strategies including leaflets distributed in health centres and billboards erected along major highways and in public spaces such as transport yards, markets, hospital car parks and sports grounds. They joined billboards and signposts sponsored by other international and national organizations such as Ghana AIDS Commission and Family Health International (Figure 4.1) and smaller signposts commissioned by local organisations (Figure 4.2). Cumulatively, they contributed to a 'transnational imagescape' (Quayson, 2014) of HIV/AIDS. Along the major highways criss-crossing the country, some of these billboards remain in their original locations, colours and texts faded, decades after they were erected.

The SALL mass media strategy was complemented by a community-centred stigma reduction programme, called Reach Out Show Compassion (hereafter ROSC), which engaged religious leaders in HIV/AIDS advocacy. Boulay and colleagues (2008) describe the process:

> local religious leaders received training on HIV/AIDS counselling, care and support, and on the importance of stigma reduction and compassion for people affected by HIV or AIDS. They were provided with posters and

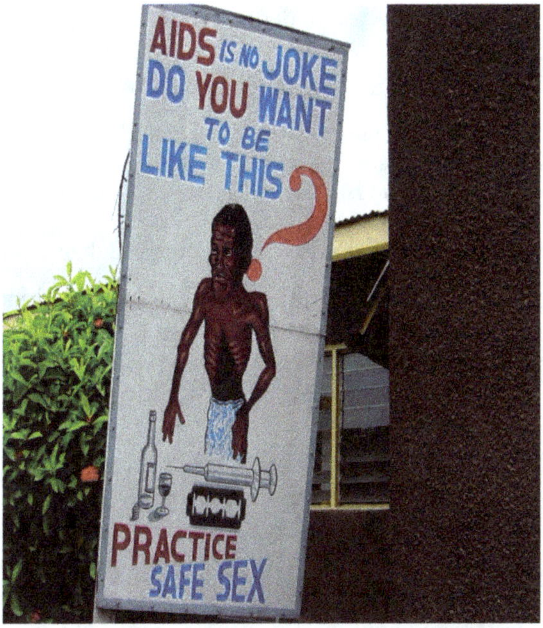
AIDS IS NO JOKE
DO YOU WANT TO BE LIKE THIS?
PRACTICE SAFE SEX

Figure 4.2 'Do you want to be like this?' Signpost outside a local clinic in Obuasi.

> other print materials to display within their church or mosque, were encouraged to incorporate themes related to compassion for PLHA in their sermons and to initiate discussions within their congregations, and they were provided with a toolkit of group activities that they could implement within their congregation (p.134).

Short video documentaries were produced of the engagement process. These videos were broadcast on national television and distributed to faith-based organisations and community-based organisations working with religious groups.

The SALL mass media campaign, along with campaigns organised by other donor institutions, created awareness of HIV/AIDS across the country. But near universal awareness did not translate to universal protective behaviours or stigma reduction. Boulay and colleagues (2008) analysed the effectiveness of the ROSC strategy of using religious leaders to reduce HIV-related stigma. Two surveys were conducted in the Greater Accra, Ashanti and Upper East regions: a baseline survey conducted in 2001 with 2,746 people a year before the intervention with religious leaders was implemented; a follow-up survey conducted in 2003 with 2,926 people a year after the intervention. Respondents were male and female youth and adults aged between 15 and 59.

The surveys explored three stigma related questions:

> 1) if a member of your family got infected with the virus that cause AIDS, would you want it to remain a secret?; 2) if a relative of yours became sick with the virus that causes AIDS, would you be willing to care for him or her in your own household?; and, 3) If a female teacher has the virus that causes AIDS, should she be allowed to continue teaching the school?[4] (p.135).

Messages disseminated via broadcast media (television and radio) reached the greatest number of respondents. This was followed by messages on posters and billboards. Messages disseminated via programme-related community events and during religious services reached a very limited number of respondents.

Favourable attitudes towards people living with HIV/AIDS improved slightly between the baseline and follow-up periods and these were positively associated with respondents' exposure to the campaign. But there was no change in attitudes to secrecy between the two survey periods. Bouley and colleagues reported that these attitudes were influenced by the new knowledge disseminated via the ROSC campaigns as well as social norms and perceptions of risk. But they offered a partial explanation on why attitudes to secrecy and blame did not change:

> although the reasons for this selective effect are not entirely clear, it may illustrate that individuals link compassion with the alleviation of suffering. The campaign's emphasis on the theme of compassion may have prompted individuals to reconsider additional punishments for people already suffering from HIV infection, regardless of whether or not they blamed these individuals for their infection (p.139).

HIV/AIDS was considered a deadly disease during the SALL campaign period. The idea and image of the condition evoked complicated emotions of fear, distrust, disgust, shame and denial, which drove stigmatising practices. Therefore, one could feel compassion for a relative with HIV, and still want to keep their status a secret to prevent courtesy stigma. Secondly, secrecy is a dominant cultural strategy for processing illness, especially with the category of 'bought diseases' that are attributed to social

[4] UNAIDS reported that 11,000 of 2.4 million primary school children had lost a teacher to AIDS in 1999 (Vanderpuye and Amegatcher, 2004). This statistic did not suggest that female teachers were at greater risk.

and spiritual causes, as we saw with Ruth's story in Chapter 2 and will see in family stories later in this chapter.

Crucially, the SALL campaign itself reinforced negative mixed emotions that undermined its message of compassion. First, the campaign song applied a fear appeal approach which has had mixed to no impact in health promotion campaigns around the world for a range of behaviours including dental hygiene, anti-smoking, seat-belt wearing and safe sex (Campbell, 2003; Job, 1988; Kok et al., 2018). Critical health psychologists argue that fear elicits a distancing effect from health-enabling behaviour, rather than a pull towards changing health-disabling behaviours. Furthermore, in contexts where there are no enabling environments to support new health habits, people are unlikely to adopt them. In Ghana, public health experts blamed poor responses to HIV/AIDS educational interventions on a prevailing attitude of 'all die be die': "a statement that translates to 'every death is death', implying that each person is going to die and that the cause of death does not matter much" (Awusabo-Asare et al., 1999, p.125). In poor and marginalised communities where decades of structural neglect had created overwhelming developmental and health problems, illness was the new figure, health the ground. Forged in these contexts 'all die be die' drove a tendency to underestimate health risks and to ignore or deny illness. This tendency also blurred cultural distinctions between good death (which "comes 'naturally' after a long and well spent life") and bad death (which comes unnaturally and prematurely) (van der Geest, 2004, p.899). Fear appeals did not work for recipients who were not afraid of death or dying through stigmatising circumstances. In actual fact, despite the SALL song's fear appeal, the line 'it's not on, it's not in' became a humorous catch phrase in popular culture.[5]

Second, the visuals that accompanied the campaign, projected HIV largely through the tropes of severe sickness and of death and dying. Social psychological theories of knowledge production, such as social representations theory (Moscovici and Duveen, 2001), propose that individuals and communities construct new knowledge through the processes of anchoring and objectification. Anchoring occurs when unfamiliar phenomena or ideas are classified and named, by setting them in a familiar context of pre-existing knowledge systems. Objectification is the process through which unfamiliar phenomena or ideas are condensed into a 'figurative nucleus' – "a complex of images that visibly reproduces a

[5] See for example Episode 30 of TWDFL on YouTube (www.youtube.com/watch?v=cLYU706DMus).

complex of ideas" (Moscovici, 1984, p.29). Objectification reproduces the unfamiliar 'among the things we can see and touch and thus control' (Moscovici, 1984, p.29) or as Sandra Jovchelovitch (2001, p.172) succinctly describes, gives "novelty a concrete, almost 'natural' face". Once unfamiliar phenomena are linked to a figurative nucleus, this joins other images circulating in the symbolic social environment and in social imaginaries, becomes a subject of communication, a constituent of social practices, and the (re)construction of reality.[6] By 2001, as we saw in Chapter 2, HIV/AIDS had become 'the natural face' of conditions, such as uncontrolled diabetes, that came with sudden and/or sustained weight loss. Through community speculation, gossip and distancing, individuals living with these conditions experienced inadvertent HIV/AIDS discrimination and stigma (de-Graft Aikins, 2006). Transnational imagescapes of HIV/AIDS projected new ways of anchoring and objectifying disease into national consciousness and social imaginaries that continue to shape social attitudes to serious illness today.

'Even Snakes Like Music': Folk Media

The second popular arts-based approach to HIV/AIDS prevention was through the use of 'folk media'. Solomon Panford and colleagues (2001) define 'folk media' as "traditional forms of communication [that] have evolved as grassroots expressions of the values and lifestyles of the people and because they use local languages . . . have become embedded in their cultural, social and psychologic thinking" (p.1560). Their list of folk media includes a combination of traditional arts and popular arts discussed in previous chapters: "storytelling, puppetry, proverbs, visual art, drama, role-play, concerts, gong beating, dirges, songs, drumming and dancing" (p.1560).

During the early years of the pandemic musicians, choral groups and community members composed HIV prevention songs of their own accord or in response to official competitions for songs. HIV/AIDS songs were composed in five genres – Highlife, Hiplife, Gospel, Choral music and Dirges. Kofi Poku Quan-Baffour (2007) presents examples of each genre in his brief review of the use of folk media in HIV/AIDS education, highlighting the production of these songs by famous musicians – Highlife icon Nana Kwame Ampadu, and Gospel singer McAbraham – as well as local singing

[6] Moscovici has argued that: "when an image linked to a word or idea becomes detached and is let loose in a society it is accepted as a reality" (Moscovici, 1984, p.39).

groups such as *Black Bugu and Sika Nti Mmrante*. Angela Scharfenberger (2011) documents two songs – *HIV Is Real* and *We Are True* – composed by the Young and Wise Inspirational Choir, an Accra-based youth choir, with members aged fourteen to twenty. The choir was supported by the Planned Parenthood Association of Ghana (PPAG), which also supported a women's choir, a drama group and a cultural group, through five Young and Wise Centres it established in Accra and other cities.

These 'unofficial' HIV songs focused on prevention through fear appeals and morality tales. Played on radio, on street sound systems, at faith gatherings and in other public spaces, they complemented the official mass media campaign songs.

The second type of folk media was applied theatre. Panford and colleagues (2001) presented basic outlines of applied theatre projects piloted in rural areas in the Ashanti Region, including the participatory live shows produced by Theatre for Communication Implementation and Development (Theatre CID), a local group based in Kumasi, which educated "curious crowds about pertinent health issues, such as family planning, breast-feeding and HIV/AIDS" (p.1561). Kwardua Vanderpuye and Janet Amegatcher (2004) described a pilot project conducted in Accra in January 2002 with 900 youth aged between twelve and twenty-three, associated with International Youth Shelter Foundation Ghana. The project applied the 'forum theatre' approach pioneered by Brazilian theatre practitioner Augusto Boal, as a data collection method to examine youth perspectives on HIV risk and infections. "Using their bodies without employing words" participants expressed "their opinion about taboo topics in the presence of adults" (p.155), including "exploitative sexual transactions between young women and 'sugar daddies'" (p.156). The topics were discussed, myths and misunderstandings were addressed and practical interventions were introduced, including condom distribution, counselling and testing and training peer educators to reinforce prevention messages. The authors emphasised the importance of involving young people in the conceptualisation and implementation of youth-focused HIV interventions.

Two projects – *The Bitter Side of AIDS* and *Asetena Pa* – used theatre as intervention in community settings. *The Bitter Side of AIDS* was an HIV/AIDS-themed play originally scripted and performed by Hewale, a theatre group set up by the MOH to dramatize AIDS messages to communities, workplaces and faith-based spaces in Accra. The success of the Accra production inspired the MOH to fund performances for other communities in the Ashanti and Eastern regions. Kwadwo Bosompra (2007–2008) led a research project undertaken by the MOH's Health

Education Division to evaluate the impact of the play, after it was performed to communities in urban Koforidua and rural Konko, in the Eastern Region. The play told a story about a woman who gave birth to an HIV-positive baby. The infection was traced, not to the woman's husband and father of her baby but, to her former sexual partner.

Bosompra's evaluation applied focus group discussions to examine community engagement and understandings of the play, as well as popular AIDS songs. Between 112 and 168 community members were recruited for the focus group study. Eight groups were convened in urban Koforidua and six groups in rural Konko. The groups were segmented along age (adult, youth) and gender (male, female). Half of the FGD participants had watched the play; half had not. Groups were convened one day after the play was performed, and one month afterwards. The two sets of discussions yielded four insights.

First, the theatrical production worked. Community members remembered the central story and found it credible. The actors were praised for their realistic portrayal of the story. More importantly participants shared the story and its insights to significant others – spouses, partners, parents, siblings and children.

Secondly, it was evident that national mass media campaigns on HIV/AIDS prevention, folk media messaging and broader public perceptions of HIV/AIDS had filtered through to both communities, via mass media and family and social networks. Radio was an especially powerful medium. When community members were asked about AIDS songs they had heard, Nana Kwame Ampadu's *AIDS Nnye* was on the top of the list. Ampadu's song received as much radio airplay as the SALL song, tackled the same ABC themes as SALL, and used fear appeals. Most people heard *AIDS Nnye* on radio; others heard the song from children who memorised and sang it as they played in their local neighbourhoods.

Yare bi aba eye owuo	A certain disease has come, it is death
Yare de AIDS ooh	The disease is AIDS ooh
AIDS anaa,	It is AIDS
Yare bi aba enni aduro	A certain disease has come, it has no cure
Enya wo a ebeku wo	If it gets you, it will kill you
Enti amanfo mo ma yemo ye ho ban	So people, let's protect ourselves
Eye a hye roba ana AIDS annye wo	Wear a condom, so you don't get AIDS

(source: Quan-Baffour, 2007)

In addition to songs, community members were familiar with HIV/AIDS cures promoted by indigenous healers. Kwaku Fri, a shrine priest based in Nwoase, in the Brong Ahafo (Bono East) region, emerged as an influential source of information on HIV/AIDS treatment and cures. His messages were disseminated via television and radio.

> A fetish priest, Kwaku Firi, in Brong Ahafo has got a cure. It is shown on TV a lot of times and he has cured many people.
>
> It was on the TV; there was this traditional African priest with a man and a woman he had cured and who had been proved to be cured at Korle-Bu Teaching Hospital.

Thirdly, community members knew what worked for them in relation to arts-based health communication. They wanted nuanced visuals. Some wanted to see what a baby with HIV infection looked like and the trajectory of HIV infection: "the play should be able to show the signs of the disease on those who had it" (p.141). They wanted multi-form arts. Some preferred 'plays that were preceded by music and dancing' (p.141). There was a consensus that music was an important conduit for HIV/AIDS education: "even snakes like music" (p.147) as one participant memorably asserted. The popular HIV/AIDS songs had 'pleasing melodies', 'danceable rhythm', were sung clearly in local languages, and contained sound advice (p.145). But a number of community members pointed out there had to be a balance between entertaining and educating: when "the music is too beautiful, it makes you shake to the beat instead of listening to the words" (p.146). Even when the words were listened to, the message could be difficult to implement. For example, while most people appreciated the sound advice contained in the popular songs, the ABC messages had mixed impact for sexually active young men and women in casual relationships. Young men struggled with the advice on wearing condoms; some struggled to 'be faithful' to one partner.[7] Young women struggled with negotiating safe sex.

Finally, community members knew what their pressing health problems were. While HIV/AIDS was perceived as a serious health threat at the national level and urban (Koforidua) level, rural community members did not believe this was the dominant problem for them. Both urban and rural communities outlined a range of health and development concerns that they believed to be more, or as equally, important as HIV/AIDS. Urban groups listed guinea worm infection, kwashiorkor, malaria and lack of

[7] Similar sentiments were expressed in a study by Catherine MacPhail and Catherine Campbell (2001) on condom wearing among young South Africans aged thirteen to twenty-five: "I think condoms are good but, aai, I hate those things".

potable water. Rural groups listed guinea worm infection and the lack of biomedical facilities.

The *Asetena Pa* (The Good Life, in Twi) Project, documented by Gail Boneh and Devan Jaganeth Jaganath (2011), applied the concert party approach to "empower people with HIV/AIDS and initiate a public discourse on HIV/AIDS that includes structural and contextual issues" (p.458).

The concert party is an indigenous Ghanaian multi-arts theatrical tradition that was developed in Fante coastal towns in the 1910s (Collins, 1976). Theatrical productions blended music, dance and comedy, drawing influences from traditional Akan folklore, in particular *Anansesem* (spider stories) (Dakubu, 1990), as well as imported entertainment forms from Europe and North America, such as sea shanties, vaudeville, 'Black American ragtimes' and ballroom dances like the foxtrot (Collins, 1976). During the early decades performances catered to elite urban audiences; then the focus shifted to 'newly arrived rural immigrants' to major cities in the south. As popular culture expanded between the 1950s to 1970s to include music from the Caribbean (such as calypso) and other parts of Africa (such as Afrobeat pioneered by Nigerian icon Fela Ransome Kuti), these new forms were incorporated into the repertoires of traveling theatre groups who performed to urban and rural audiences. Present-day performances continue to target diverse populations through community events across the country and through televised shows. A typical production begins with a few hours of music, dance and comedy to whip up the crowd. The play is interactive, with audience members encouraged to comment on and intervene in storylines and the trajectories of characters. Throughout its century-long evolution, the concert party has performed multiple functions, including releasing psychosocial tension through participatory comedy and physical performance, educating audiences by incorporating new socio-cultural and political trends in storylines and, in some cases, catalysing grassroots movement for social change (Collins, 1976, 2017). In this sense, the concert party bears a close resemblance – in structure and goals – to prominent applied theatre approaches, such as Augusto Boal's forum theatre, that builds on audience participation ('spect-actors'), and uses theatre to entertain, educate and challenge oppressive social structures.[8]

[8] Maria Stuttaford and colleagues (2006, p.35) capture Boal's (1992) description of Forum Theatre: "at no time should an idea be imposed. Forum Theatre does not preach, it is not dogmatic, it does not seek to manipulate people. At best, it liberates the spect-actors. At best, it stimulates them. At best, it transforms them into actors. Actor – he or she who acts."

The *Asetena Pa* story centred on a young HIV positive widow whose husband had died of AIDS and who faced a dilemma of disclosing her status to a new suitor. Unlike *The Bitter Side*, this play was scripted through a participatory process, by a group of ten professional and amateur actors, half of whom lived with HIV. The play was performed to young audiences (aged sixteen to thirty-five) in four towns in the Northern Region: Yapei, Damongo, Bole and Bamboi. In the concert party tradition, each performance began with two hours of music and comedy. Audience views were sought after the play was performed, and through focus group discussions with a selection of audience members a day after the performance.

The presence of people with HIV/AIDS on the stage who looked healthy and projected strength and confidence – presented a powerful image that contrasted the public perception of the sick and dying AIDS patient. Watching the theatre production and engaging with the actors, including actors living with HIV, empowered some individuals to test their status, to join patient support groups and to form support groups of their own. Discussions about the structural context of HIV revealed lay concerns about gendered and class-based differences in HIV experience and the oppressive impact of stigma.[9] Among the actors living with HIV, women were less likely to disclose their status due to disproportionate stigmatisation of women in Ghanaian society.

The Asetena Pa method demonstrated how lived experiences of HIV could be presented authentically and powerfully, through theatre, to galvanise empowered action at personal and group levels in Northern communities. A key limitation, the authors reported, was a lack of funding to support the transformation of personal and relational empowerment to collective empowerment and community change.

'*Ahokyer Yarba*' (A Disease of Stress): Lived Experiences

Yankah (2004) conducted narrative interviews with individuals living with HIV/AIDS and their caregivers in Accra and undisclosed locations. Data collection started in 1987, one year after the first cases of HIV infection were reported in the country, and before public health education on AIDS was fully established across the country. Data collection ended in 2003 when public education had gained considerable ground. In the early years HIV was referred to, euphemistically in some Fante communities, as

[9] The gendered dimensions of stigma, were reinforced in the imagery and content of mass media campaigns, see Caroline Faria (2008).

'*ahokyer yarba*' (a disease of stress, a version of *asetamu yareɛ* discussed in Chapter 2). Yankah was interested in what he referred to as AIDSLore: "all folk practices and interactions that are generated by the AIDS pandemic" (p.197). He was also interested in how "verbal taboos, or the notion of the unspeakable" shaped folk constructions of the disease and its spread and perceptions of risk and vulnerability. Yankah presented life stories of five adult men and women who lived with AIDS. They had all migrated to other West African countries, where they had contracted AIDS.

Abeku was forty years old. When Yankah first spoke to him he had been an in-patient at the Korle-Bu teaching hospital for two weeks. Abeku went to Cote d'Ivoire with his wife, leaving his children behind. He contracted HIV in Cote d'Ivoire and he believed his use of Ghanaian sex workers, during his wife's trips to Ghana, might have led to his illness. He never mentioned AIDS by name. A non-disclosure policy operating at the hospital appeared to amplify his strategy of denial. His doctor had not named the disease. A nurse claimed: "we are not supposed to tell the patient or his relatives; that's not our duty. Most of the patients think it's cholera they have, because of the vomiting and diarrhoea involved" (p.187).[10]

Mama was forty years old. She had just had a baby and been discharged from Korle-Bu when she was first interviewed. Mama had also migrated to Cote d'Ivoire to make a living to cater for the nine children she had left behind. Their father did not provide for them. She had spent four months healer-shopping for a cure for her infection before returning to Ghana.

Solo, a man in his fifties, had recently returned from Nigeria. Yankah interviewed his father, an eighty-four year-old retired teacher who narrated a story of loss and regret. Solo had worked for a rich Nigerian for years, he lived a 'high life' in a 'big mansion' and 'ate well'. But he had been estranged from his family in Ghana, including three children he left behind. When Solo got sick, he sought diagnosis and treatment from clinics and shrines in Nigeria. After failed attempts to secure healing, he came home to spend his final days with his father.

Yaa was forty-two years old. Her story was narrated by a cousin, who lived in their family household. She had grown lean and weak and could

[10] This strategy of non-disclosure at the Korle-Bu Teaching Hospital, was reported in other African countries. Nguyen (2010, p.21) describes a silent hospital non-disclosure policy in Burkina Faso, in the early years of the pandemic: "HIV-testing were rarely available, and even if they were, patients were still not told of their diagnosis. Winston, a nurse in one of the main medical wards... gave a simple reason for not informing the patients: "Patients aren't told because it would only discourage them ... once an HIV patient gets transferred to the chronic section, he realizes that he has HIV even if he hasn't been told, and he rarely lasts more than a few days."

not walk without help. Yaa's younger sister had died of AIDS at age thirty-five. Although her symptoms were recognised as AIDS by her family, Yaa did not believe she had AIDS. One day, Yaa left home at dawn and never came back. Many household members believed she had left in order to spare her mother the shame of a bad death.

Auntie B, age unknown, died from AIDS. She may have contracted HIV from her husband who also died of AIDS a few years prior.

Yankah's respondents attributed HIV/AIDS to physical, social and spiritual causes. Spiritual causal theories were dominant and weaved through the other explanations – in similar ways to diabetes causal theories in Nkoranza (Chapter 2).

Two days before Yaa was diagnosed with HIV, she had a dream that she had been given 'spiritual meat'.

> She said she dreamed that somebody, a woman, had given her something like spiritual meat to eat. The disease started two days after the dream (p.194).

Although Solo's father understood he had AIDS, he believed the illness and his son's eventual death was driven by spiritual factors: "the doctor had told him it was not a dangerous cough. But it was incurable. It has to be spiritual" (p.193). Auntie B's family believed her husband was 'spiritually killed by a Nigerian wholesaler' to whom he owed money (p.195).

Across the country AIDS cures and stigma protection charms were offered by herbalists, 'spiritualists' and shrine priests who advertised on mass media (television, radio, newspapers) and in public spaces (via signposts, verbal adverts on public transport and spaces). Shrine priests in Brong Ahafo region encountered earlier in the narratives of people in Koforidua and Konko, and in Chapter 2, emerged again as the masters in selling AIDS cures. Yankah quoted a 2003 article in the Mirror, one of Ghana's national newspapers:

> Relatives of HIV/AIDS patients in the Brong Ahafo region are said to be paying large sums of money to powerful shrine keepers to protect their families from the stigma of the disease. The shrine keepers usually demand huge sums of money, and items like cement, roofing sheets, and some bottles of schnapps from willing relatives, and in turn protect AIDS victims from being stigmatized, by claiming that the gods have cursed the patients (p.196).

Most respondents blended biomedical treatment with traditional healing. Like community members in Koforidua and Konko, they got their information on HIV and HIV treatment choices from the mass media, radio in particular, and from family and friends.

Yaa visited a spiritualist who declared the woman in the dream she had two days before her diagnosis was her mother. The spiritualist did not appear to prescribe a treatment that worked.

> She then went to a spiritualist, who invited her mother, and told her it was a spiritual disease afflicting her daughter. When her mother asked further, the spiritualist said... Yaa had been bewitched by her mother (p.194).

Before Mama returned to Ghana from Cote d'Ivoire, she visited several herbalists there. One prescribed treatment that did not work:

> I went to several herbalists, but none could help because I carried a pregnancy. One herbalist gave me herbs to boil and sit on. But each time I sat on the steam I felt the fetus turning in my womb. I realized the baby's life was in danger, so I threw the herbs away.

When Solo returned to Ghana he treated his condition at home using rituals likely obtained from a shrine priest in Nigeria:

> He probably practiced occultism, for you could tell from the power ring on his finger, and the fact that throughout the short time he spent with us, he never slept on a soft bed. He opted to sleep on leaves and newspapers, and had strange objects in his pocket, like a small bottle of water, and a tin of sardine. It looked like ritual food (p.193).

Everyday experiences within family settings were marked by complicated emotions of denial, fear and shame, but also of sustained compassion. Abeku and Yaa never accepted their HIV status. Both attributed causes to spiritual factors and not unsafe sexual behaviour. Auntie B's husband's family did not accept his HIV status, even though she contracted her infection from him. Solo's father never attributed his son's deteriorating health to HIV/AIDS. He did not ask his son probing questions: "he had told me he led a high life. But I suspect his ailment was spiritual" (p.193).

Yankah referred to these discursive strategies of "avoidance and circumvention, based on fear or embarrassment" as "a speech act – a social statement of stress" (p.197). In these family settings, where conversations and actions revolved around impending loss, there was a clear distinction between good death and bad death. The overriding attitude, to invert the popular saying, was 'all die no be die'. People did what it took to prevent a bad death (Solo's rituals), or to shield their loved ones from the stigma of a bad death in the family (Yaa's final solo journey). Indigenous healers operating in the same spaces as mass media campaigns offered diagnoses, treatments and cures for AIDS as well as mediation for the social and spiritual dimensions of the condition. In addition to biomedical treatment, individuals and their families drew on these indigenous resources from the beginning to the end of their healing journeys.

'They Stopped Playing the Songs'

Edward Maibach and colleagues (2007) observe that for health communication initiatives to create large-scale and sustained behaviour change, they must first be "heard and remembered against the din of other competing messages in the media" (p.6). Furthermore, recipients must be highly motivated to adapt the behaviour change being promoted and "few social network, group or environmental barriers should stand in the way of behaviour, and the behaviour being recommended should be easy to perform" (p.6).

Mass HIV/AIDS campaigns reached national audiences and created awareness, with songs playing an important role. But they competed with messaging from indigenous healing systems and behaviour change was modest for evaluated communities.

Folk media draws on arts traditions and established community practices. As a result songs and theatre were enjoyed, and the messages offered were accepted, remembered and shared within family and social networks. More importantly these methods offered insights into communities' knowledge about their health problems and the interventions they were likely to value: arts-based interventions had to be aligned with community preference for multi-form arts, ensure a balance between education and entertainment, and pay attention to enabling and disabling drivers of behaviour and habits.

While individuals and communities heard the HIV messaging (regardless of medium) and were motivated to reduce HIV risk, multi-layered barriers existed. Changing cultural representations of death and dying undermined fear appeals and the ABCs were difficult to adhere to, particularly for young sexually active individuals. There was also the unintended negative consequence of mass media campaigns introducing ideas and imagery which shaped harmful representations and imaginaries of serious sickness. Individuals living with HIV/AIDS encountered gendered discrimination which shaped strategies of disclosure, poor doctor–patient communication in hospital settings, and messaging from indigenous healing systems that validated spiritual causal theories, hope for cures and healing journeys. A cross-cutting problem was that none of these projects were long-term, and as one Konko resident observed in 2007, once the music stopped some communities thought HIV/AIDS had been eradicated.

In November 2021, Ivan Quashigah, the director of *TWDFL* was interviewed by the journalist Erskine Amo Whyte (also known as Rev Erskine) on YFM's MydMorning Radio Show. Whyte asked Quashigah what made *TWDFL* "such a great success". Quashigah narrated a story of serendipitous events. *TWDFL* started out as a radio series on Joy FM, and gathered an avid participatory following who lobbied for a television series. Quashigah negotiated funding for the television series in exchange for directing commercials for a women's digest show. After established writers refused to write the script for the drama, due to morality concerns, he found a willing young writer – Edward Seddoh Jnr. Character development and storylines reflected Seddoh's engagement with the realities of young people and youth culture at the time. These serendipitous events meant that even though the drama was part of the mass media campaign ecosystem at the time, it was firmly based in the folk media genre of storytelling. As a result, and in contrast to SALL and other mass media campaigns, *TWDFL* characters and storylines fired up the imagination and connected emotionally with its target audience. Long after the funding ended, the drama series lives on through YouTube viewings, reminisces and re-imaginings.

If *TWDFL* had received long-term funding, it would have joined the ranks of the African series *Shuga*, and the Miguel Sabido-pioneered Latin American soap operas with social messages, which provide key insights into how mass media drama shapes long-term behaviour change. These arts-based mass media campaigns get the balance right between contextualised breadth and depth – by focusing on evolving responses to locally relevant health problems through realistic storylines and authentic character arcs. When funded for long periods alongside structural and community-based interventions, they offer a powerful way of initiating and sustaining behaviour change over time and priming collective responses to new public health threats.

CHAPTER 5

Food Is Medicine, Food Is Poison

Edziban ah! Me le dzidzi (Ah food! Let's eat, I say!)

Fante slogan used by Kwame Dzokoto, host of the Edziban Food Show on Ghana's TV3 Television Network.

In 2006, Ghana's Ministry of Health (MOH) piloted an intervention called the Regenerative Health and Nutrition (RHN) Programme. The programme was the brainchild of the Minister of Health at the time, Major (Rtd) Courage Quashigah,[1] and was developed in collaboration with the African Hebrew Development Agency (AHDA). AHDA was established by the African Hebrew Israelite Community (AHIC), a community of African-Americans who emigrated from the south side of Chicago, via Liberia, to Dimona, Israel in the late 1960s. They lived holistic lifestyles and consumed a vegan diet, trademarked as "the Edenic Divine Diet" (Markowitz and Avieli, 2022). The Edenic Divine Diet had, "according to the community, provided numerous benefits including, the virtual elimination of lifestyle diseases (cancer, heart disease, diabetes, etc.) which plague African Americans" (Miller, 2021, p.5).

While, the community's advocacy work in the US and Israel had been well documented,[2] their leadership on the RHN programme in Ghana appeared to be the first time they had promoted their Edenic Divine Diet model to an African country through their development agency. From a development perspective, however, this unique project built on decades of African-American development work in Ghana, through the *Nkosuohene* (development chief, in Twi) initiative established by the late Asantehene

[1] Health Minister between 2001 and 2009, under the New Patriotic Party (NPP) government of President J. A Kufuor.

[2] See Markowitz and Avieli (2022). Dimona as a healing space for African-Americans was also well documented. This was famously featured in 2003 when the late superstar Whitney Houston and her husband Bobby Brown paid a 'spiritual visit' to her 'brothers and sisters in Dimona' (Houston felt 'at home' in Israel – The Jerusalem Post (jpost.com).

Otumfuo Opoku Ware II in 1985 for Asante development, and supported by successive governments since (Bob-Milliar, 2009; Guedj, 2015; McCaskie, 2009).

Major Quashigah, a former military leader, had met the community in Israel, during an official visit years prior. Their origin story and holistic lifestyle had inspired him. Quashigah was appointed health minister at a time when the rising prevalence of chronic non-communicable diseases (NCDs) such as diabetes, hypertension, strokes and cancers had become an issue of public concern. A 'double burden of malnutrition' was a risk factor in chronic diseases. This was a phenomenon whereby both overnutrition (eating high calorie foods associated with overweight and obesity) and undernutrition (eating nutrient deficient foods, or experiencing grades of starvation, associated with stunting and underweight) was present in the same community, household or individual (Popkin et al., 2019). Despite the establishment of a Non-Communicable Disease Control Programme (NCDCP) in the late 1990s, minimal progress had been made on prevention and care of chronic diseases, because the programme had been consistently understaffed and underfunded (Bosu, 2012). Between 1990 and 2010, the top twenty-five causes of premature deaths included protein energy malnutrition (which occupied a top ten position at both points of measurement) and four NCDs – stroke, diabetes, liver cancer and chronic kidney disease (de-Graft Aikins and Koram, 2017). The risk factors for conditions like stroke and diabetes include overweight and obesity. For Quashigah, the AHIC story, and in particular the community's claim to disease-free longevity, was just the innovative push that Ghanaian public health needed. The beginnings of a collaborative project was hatched then, and fine-tuned through consultative meetings between AHDA representatives and local health experts in Ghana.

The RHN programme was launched under a broad health policy theme "Our Health is our Wealth", and was piloted in nine districts in the country's (then) ten regions: Amasaman and Ada (Greater Accra), Akim-Oda (Eastern), Hohoe and Keta (Volta), Asikuma-Odobeng-Brakwa (Central), Tamale and Gushegu (Northern), Bolgatanga (Upper East) and Wa (Upper West) (see map in Appendix 1).

In each district a standard format was followed. AHDA members run a one week workshop in a local community centre. In the weeks preceding the workshop, participants were strategically selected to represent community members, community leaders, religious leaders, healthcare providers, healthcare administrators and political leaders. Workshop participants were called change agents (CAs). A training manual developed by AHDA and local experts was used in the sessions. It had three sections:

healthy lifestyles, regenerative nutrition, and child and maternal health. The Edenic Divine Diet was at the heart of the regenerative nutrition section and local recipes were re-imagined through this frame. The language of meetings was English. RHN workshop meetings began and ended with the motivational slogans: "food is medicine", "water is medicine" and "cleanliness is medicine". These slogans became RHN brands. Signposts erected outside district and community health centres provided visual reinforcement of the RHN messages. To scale up the programme to national level, Ghanaian celebrities, creative artists and media professionals were co-opted as RHN Programme advocates to share nutritional and health messages on television, radio and in public spaces. Selected RHN advocates also travelled on "study tours" to the Village of Peace, Dimona, Israel, on the government's ticket, to observe the holistic lifestyles of the African Hebrew Israelite community in situ.

The RHN programme is a rare example of a participatory health intervention in Ghana that was developed and funded by the MOH, and did not involve a dominant donor partner, such as USAID or DFID. The programme adapted a model of healthy eating that was little known in global public health, unlike the Mediterranean diet, for example. Finally, it was piloted at the community level across the country in order to develop proof of concept.[3] On paper the RHN project should have been successful and sustainable. But the pilot never matured into the national level intervention Major Quashigah envisioned. The RHN Programme has no online afterlife like *TWDFL* or SALL. What remains of the programme is the following paragraph on the MOH website, which has not been updated since it was posted in 2007:

> The Regenerative Health and Nutrition (RHN) Programme is a new preventive and promotive health care programme initiated by the Ministry of Health (MOH). It aims to transform the health, lives and socioeconomic development of Ghanaians. It is a logical policy programme after health insurance. Its long term effect can bring about a reduction in the cost of *lifestyle diseases* such as Hypertension, Diabetes, Cancer, Gout and others which are currently on the increase. *Lifestyle changes* include what people eat and drink, and their physical activity levels, rest, and cleanliness. The programme draws on the experiences of an African Hebrew Community, living in Dimona, Israel and tries to adapt them to Ghana. The main objective of the programme is to reduce the risk of

[3] Another more prominent project is the Community-based Health Planning and Services (CHPS) project. This began as a funded pilot project on task-shifting in Navrongo, Upper East Region. After successful results CHPS was scaled up across the country and has become a core plank of primary care service delivery (see Phillips et al., 2018).

> occurrence of diseases and disorders for individuals, households and communities so as to contribute to the development of a healthier and productive population that can create wealth for itself and the country (MOH website, emphasis added).

The problem of nutrition-related NCDs has intensified in the years since the programme ended, and lessons can be learned from its successes and failures. In this chapter I revisit a commissioned evaluation of the programme through the lens of its arts-based methods. The chapter unfolds in three parts. Part one outlines the evaluation methodology. Part two focuses on how the arts were used to promote the RHN core message of 'food is medicine'. While the programme promoted 'food is medicine', a competing representation of 'food is poison' prevailed across the RHN communities. This representation developed from "slow observations" (Davies, 2022) made by communities about the "slow violence" (Nixon, 2011) of toxic agricultural practices and environmental degradation. "Food is poison" undermined intentions to cook and eat more healthily. The arts could not cut through this competing message. Part three focuses on the structural determinants of the double burden of malnutrition. I consider how the cumulative impact of toxic agricultural practices, environmental degradation and food market globalisation interferes with the hybridisation of food cultures and presents conceptual and creative challenges for public health nutrition.

Evaluating the RHN Programme

In June 2007, I was commissioned by the MOH to conduct an independent review of the RHN programme. My task was to examine the impact of the programme on acceptability and behaviour change by interviewing selected change agents (CAs) in all the pilot communities, and observing their social practices and environments. I was invited to observe the final workshop, which was held in Big Ada, in the Greater Accra Region, in a community whose development chief, Nene Katey Ocansey I, was the late legendary African-American musician Isaac Hayes. With his wife, who took on the royal name of 'Princess Asie Ocansey of Ada', Hayes built the Nene Katey Ocansey I Learning and Technology (NekoTech) Center of Excellence, to support young people in the community. The NekoTech Centre hosted the workshop. The two-storey centre had meeting rooms on the ground floor where the week's sessions were held, and classrooms and offices on the first. I sat through teaching sessions, joined the Walk for Life on the beach and had the opportunity to speak to the AHDA leaders and key members about their life philosophy and their goals for the RHN programme.

Following the Big Ada experience, I spent two weeks in the field with three research assistants.[4] We had two days to gather data in each community, and so we applied a rapid appraisal method, combining interviews with observations and situated conversations, within a social psychology framework (de-Graft Aikins, 2010). We visited primary schools and talked to school children in Amasaman and Asikuma, engaged with one church congregation in Tamale, and visited a traditional birth attendant in Ho. In each community we conducted basic food surveys in one selected market and we ate in local restaurants. In Akim Oda and Keta, we were invited into the homes of CAs, for home cooked 'regenerative' meals. We bought tofu kebabs from local vendors in Akim Oda. We visited a keep-fit club in Asikuma, and in Wa met with members of a Regenerative Health Club and joined a health walk organised by a secondary school. We visited health centres in all the communities, a CHPS (Community-based Health Planning and Services) compound in Amasaman,[5] and talked to district directors of health services, district directors of nursing services and District Chief Executives (DCEs), and professionals within GHS and local government who had been tasked to support the RHN project at district level in the post-workshop phase. We interviewed 156 CAs and engaged with just over 100 people (who were not CAs) across the participating communities. Later that year, I submitted a report to the MOH, and presented key findings at a dissemination workshop convened in Ho, in the Volta Region, by the minister.

Food Is Medicine: Arts and RHN Messaging

The core RHN message – 'food is medicine' – was two-pronged: "eat more locally grown foods and vegetables" and "avoid processed foods". This dual message was emphasised during the workshops. Eat locally produced brown rice, instead of imported white rice; cook with local spices such as black peppercorns and basil, instead of processed bouillon cubes such as Nestle's Maggi cubes and Unilever's Royco cubes; drink teas made from local herbs such as moringa, instead of instant coffee with tinned milk. There was also a major emphasis on cutting back on meat and eating more soya protein and tofu. This message was promoted through slogans and

[4] In the first five districts (Amasaman, Asikuma, Tamale, Gushegu and Wa) the research assistant was Macarius Donneyong, in the sixth district (Bolgatanga) the research assistant was Edward Adiiboka, and in the final four (Akim Oda, Hohoe, Keta and Ada) the research assistant was Kobina Abaka Ansah. Donneyong was a graduate nutritionist, Adiiboka and Ansah were graduate demographers.

[5] See Phillips et al. (2018).

signposts, a celebrity campaign, and traditional recipes re-imagined through the Divine Edenic Diet.

Slogans and Signposts

Verbal and written slogans are ubiquitous in Ghanaian social life, as we saw in Chapter 2. The RHN project built on this social practice to some measurable effect. In Big Ada, lessons were punctuated with call and response interludes. Instructors would call out "regenerative health", and workshop participants would respond "renew your strength, prevent disease". These slogans were reproduced on signposts, along with other core RHN messages including eating more locally grown staples, drinking water, engaging in physical activity and avoiding processed foods. RHN signposts had a simple text-based design. A branded logo of three figures with raised hands in red, yellow, green and black (colours chosen to reflect the colours of Ghana's flag), was situated at the top. Below this, text in blue and red alternating lines were crammed onto a white background. Some signposts added blocks of colour to accentuate selected texts, others did not. Signposts were placed in strategic locations on the grounds of healthcare centres (Figure 5.1).

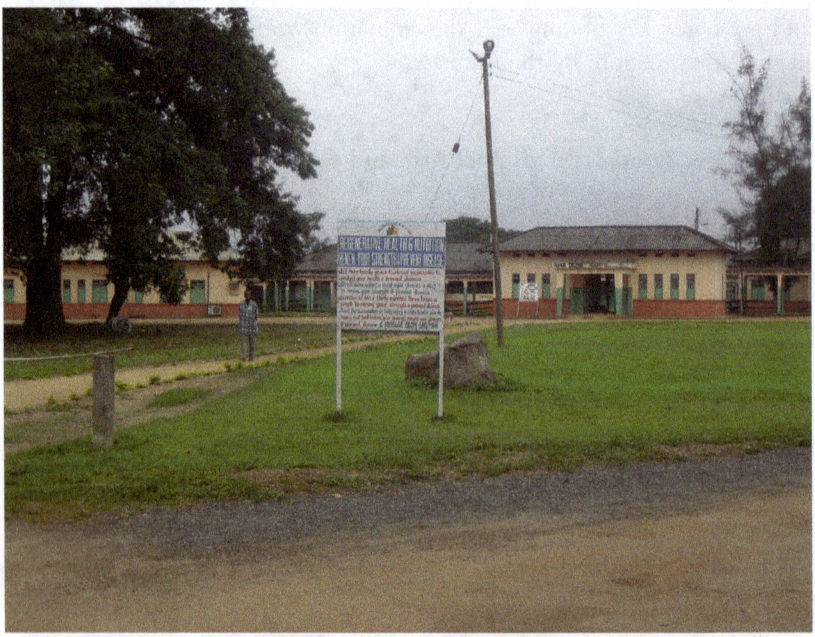

Figure 5.1 RHN signpost outside Hohoe District Hospital, Volta Region.

The core dietary messages were remembered months after the initial RHN workshops. In communities where RHN clubs had been established and met regularly (such as in Wa), the ritual of starting meetings and punctuating sessions with the slogans amplified the message for club members. Some CAs had shared the core RHN message with family members and significant others who did not participate in the workshops. The signposts placed outside selected local clinics and district hospitals reinforced the core messages of RHN for community members who used these facilities. Although workshop participants were selected based on English language proficiency, a few evaluation participants criticized the over-reliance on English language as the dominant language of instruction during the workshop and for branded project activities.

The Celebrity Campaign

The RHN programme adapted lessons from previous mass media health campaigns, such as SALL, by involving celebrities in the amplification of the RHN messages. One prominent Accra-based radio host, Abeiku Santana, incorporated RHN messages into his daily shows. For a short period, the programme leaders attempted to sign on Gyedu-Blay Ambolley, Ghana's highlife icon and a long-time vegan (who was also a member of Ghana All Stars, see Chapter 4), as a key spokesperson for the programme. He spoke once, at a food fair held at the premises of the MOH headquarters in Accra. There were no follow-up activities with him after this. Few CAs mentioned celebrities associated with RHN. The celebrity campaigns did not appear to have had an impact, largely because the messaging was concentrated in Accra. It is also likely the campaign did not work because apart from Abeiku Santana, none of the advocates seemed to have paid their end of the bargain after they returned from their study tour to Dimona.[6]

Re-Imagining Traditional Recipes through the Edenic Divine Diet

At the core of the programme was a set of new recipes that built on existing local cuisines. In Big Ada, I observed cooking demonstrations that focused on re-creating local recipes and meals with healthier ingredients, healthier ways of cooking (e.g. steaming instead of deep frying) and the use of soya protein and tofu as meat substitutes. These recipes were also set as cookery

[6] In Accra-based research and policy communities, the Dimona Study Tour was perceived as a project of patronage which privileged public figures with close relationships to the Minister and his team.

homework for participants. Ingredients for these new "fortified Ghanaian recipes" were provided in an appendix to the training manual, with the message "prepare these dishes according to local traditions without meat and enjoy the taste!" (MOH, 2012, p. 82). The recipes included "Palmnut soup & fufu with baked tofu", "Apem & greens with tofu or agushi", "banku & fresh pepper with battered tofu or roast" and "okro sauce baked with tofu or gluten" (MOH, 2012, pp.82–83).

The new recipes had a mixed impact. The active adoption of regenerative meals occurred in a small group of women. In Tamale, Wa, Akim-Oda, Keta and Ada, CAs reported adding soya protein to stews and soups. In Keta, CAs cooked brown rice occasionally. In Akim-Oda and Ada, CAs avoided bouillon cubes and other artificial spices and incorporated local spices in their dishes. In Amasaman, Hohoe, Keta, and Ada, moringa had become a herb of choice for teas and as food seasoning. In these districts some CAs had even planted moringa trees in their gardens. In Akim Oda some women cooked and sold regenerative meals and snacks for profit, or for official district health committee events.

There were challenges to adopting regenerative nutrition diets. Most CAs noted that insufficient time was allocated to the demonstration sessions to enable CAs to gain practical experience in making new food products such as soya milk and soya kebabs. Secondly, the basic ingredients required to make these products were either unavailable or very expensive. The CA who served us a tofu-based tomato stew with local brown rice in Keta did not cook this meal often, she told us, because the cost was prohibitive, and making tofu from scratch was time-consuming.

The new recipes did not catch on beyond this small group of CAs, because the programme did not factor in the complexity of local cuisines and food cultures. The programme also ignored a shared concern about the toxicity of staple foods and the encroaching power of cheaper imported processed foods.

'Giving up Meat Will Not Happen in Ghana'

In food studies, recipes have been described as 'culinary texts' or 'living transcripts of daily cooking' (McCann, 2010). The cooking process itself is seen as an art form.[7] Recipes and cooking provide insights into continuities and changes in local cuisines. Rose Omari and colleagues (2013, p.30) list

[7] Among the LoDagaa in northwestern Ghana, cooking, the domain of women, required knowledge which translated in the local Dagaree language "*nooro be nooro*", *as*: "working their wonders" (McCann, 2010, p.130).

four intersecting characteristics of the 'cuisine concept': "(1) "basic food" or primary "edibles"; (2) distinct techniques of preparing food; (3) distinct "flavour principle"; and (4) a set of manners and codes of etiquette". I will discuss these ideas through one traditional recipe that was targeted for culinary re-imagination by the RHN experts: 'palmnut soup and fufu'.

There is a popular saying often attributed to Asante communities that is captured in an interview between American food studies scholar Fran Osseo-Asare and the Ghanaian cookbook author Dinah Ayensu.[8]

> There are people who'll say they haven't eaten the whole day, simply because they haven't had their soup and fufu. If you give them anything – bread sandwich, Caesar salad – they don't consider it as food, until they've sat down with their bowl of fufu and soup (cited in Williams-Forson, 2014, p. 69).

In *Onions are my Husband*, an anthropological study of market women in Kumasi, American anthropologist Gracia Clark (1994), described the way Asante market women built their work routines, including the hiring of assistants and organisation of childcare, around the preparation of fufu and soup – 'the only completely satisfying food' (p.349) – for their families.

Fufu is a form of dumpling made by peeling, boiling and pounding – in a large wooden mortar with a long wooden pestle – individual, or a combination of, starchy foods like plantain, cassava and yam. There is an art to preparation, as Clark (1994) describes: "pounding fufu requires strength and coordination, turning the lump in rhythm between each stroke of the pestle and reaching each family member's preferred soft or hard consistency" (p.351). Fufu belongs to a category of 'swallow foods' (Haleegoah et al., 2016) and is eaten, with the (right) hand, with a variety of soups.

Fufu and palm nut soup (*abenkwan*, in Twi), in particular, is a major meal not only for Asante communities, but also for other Akan groups. The meal appears in folktales, children's songs and popular music.[9] Palm nut soup on its own has ritual significance for several ethnic groups. It is a soup of choice for lactating mothers, because it is believed to improve breast milk production (de-Graft Aikins, 2011). It is the accompaniment of choice for *kpopkoi*, the meal used to memorialise ancestors and propitiate the gods during the Ga Homowo festival.

[8] Dinah Ayensu is reported to have authored the first Ghanaian cookbook in 1972 – titled The Art of West African Cooking – for a foreign readership.

[9] See the popular Fante children's song *Pete Pete* (Vulture Vulture) in Appendix 3.

The core ingredients are tomatoes, onions, chilli peppers, palm fruit, meat, fish and shellfish. Salt, spices and vegetables like okra, eggplant and mushrooms are added for taste, as a garnish or accompaniment. These ingredients and the cooking process differ slightly across ethnic groups. As food systems have changed at home, and Ghanaians living abroad have improvised with new ingredients, further culinary adjustments have been made (Adjonyoh, 2017; Osseo-Asare and Baeta, 2015; Renne, 2007; Tuomainen, 2009; Williams-Forson, 2014). Busy cooks use cans of processed cream of palm fruit, instead of preparing from scratch – a multi-stage process that involves boiling and pounding the nuts to extract the cream. Canned plum tomatoes can replace fresh tomatoes. In wealthy homes, tomatoes, vegetables, chillies and spices can be blended in food processors instead of stone grinders or earthenware grinding pots. The fufu itself can be prepared from processed plantain, casava and yam flour: blended with water, brought to boil and kneaded with a spatula into a dumpling. Cooking what Ghanaians call 'neat fufu' reduces preparation time and removes the need for a cook's assistant.[10]

In the RHN updated recipe, the fufu-making process remained the same, but the preparation of soup was modified. Instead of meat and fish, added at the early stages of cooking baked tofu was added at the end of the cooking process. Extra time had to be allocated to make the tofu – and the nature of soups meant one had to take particular care with its texture. One can argue that adding tofu is an acceptable culinary innovation – it involves adding a processed food ingredient in the same way that processed cream of palm fruit is substituted for homemade pulp, or canned peeled plum tomatoes replace fresh tomatoes. But it is innovation towards a culinary cul-de-sac.

Cooking palm nut soup is a lengthy and laborious process, taking up to 3 hours depending on the approach. But the process is multi-sensory. Each stage releases layers of smells of spices, steamed meats and fish, and overtones of the palm fruit as ingredients cook through. Learning how to make palm nut soup correctly, with all the ingredients cooked in the correct way, is a rights-of-passage for young Ghanaian girls. While the recipe differs across ethnic groups, and for Ghanaian communities abroad, core aspects remain the same. Meats and fish lie at the heart of an authentic palm nut soup: this is what gives the soup its signature flavour

[10] In *Zoe's Ghana Kitchen*, the British chef Zoe Adjonyoh (2017) speaks for the younger urban and diaspora Ghanaian generation when she exclaims: "The strength and stamina required to make fufu from scratch could put it into an Olympic sporting category! If you ever get the chance, I do recommend having a go, but all-hail packet fufu for a simpler life!" (p.173).

and taste. Adding tofu does not only change the core identity of the soup, it also changes the cuisine itself: smells change, and there is a marked difference in touch and taste.

Culturally, therefore, the idea of baked tofu replacing meat in palm nut soup would be unimaginable in a Ghanaian household – whether Asante or not – for whoever cooks or eats the dish. For the majority of CAs, this was one reason for shunning the tofu-based recipes: "giving up meat will not happen in Ghana" or "Ghanaians love their meat too much" were some opinions. The second reason was closely associated with the first. For people who ate their meals in public spaces, such as chop bars, where all eyes and ears were trained on the loudly transacted ordering process, one risked being labelled poor by ordering soup without meat. Many did not want the stigma of a diminished social status and explicitly sought to avoid it. One young man in Asikuma recounted his experience:

> one of the challenges is that when I go the. . .chop bar, I used to buy food without buying meat and some would think I don't have money, so people used to laugh at me. People buy fufu with too much meat and they think it shows wealth, meanwhile they don't know they are reducing their age. So sometimes I tell them that what you people are eating is not good. . . my own is good, but they would laugh at me. Always they thought I didn't have money to buy the meat. That is the challenge I have.

His friend, another young man, declared: "nobody wants to be called a miser".

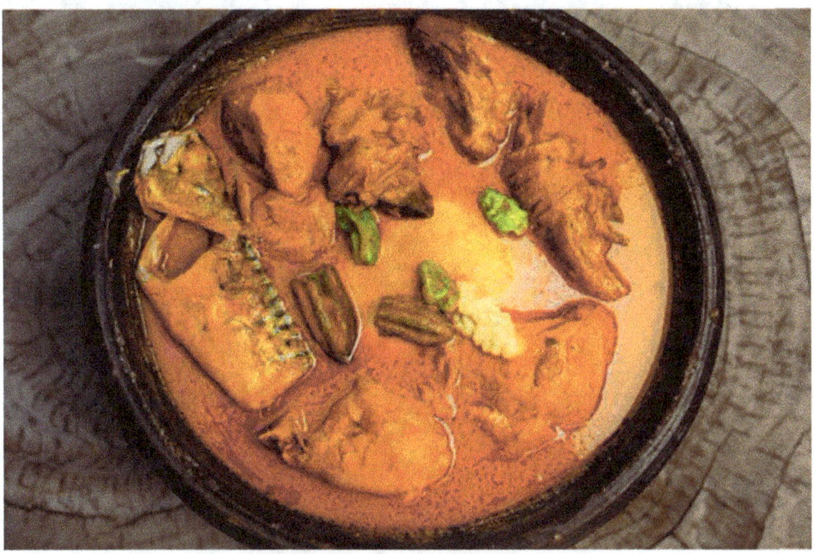

Figure 5.2 A bowl of fufu and palmnut soup.

"We Are Afraid of the Chemicals"

In addition to the problem of unavailable and expensive regenerative foods, participants also expressed grave concerns about the impact of toxic agricultural practices and environmental degradation on staple foods. CAs in most districts expressed misgivings about eating fresh vegetables and fruit because of fears of contamination.

> the bananas they are selling here. . .if you eat it, it is like you have taken pills in your mouth, as if they have forced it to ripe[en]. . .now they are spraying them too so we are afraid of the chemicals, and the vegetables too now, the okro, garden eggs, even the pepper too, they are spraying everything. *So during the workshop some asked that question. . .that they would like to take the fruit, but. . .what would happen to them because they are using a lot of chemicals* (young female community nurse, Amasaman, emphasis added).

Ultra-processed unhealthy foods were abundant, often cheaper and aggressively advertised in all the RHN recipient communities. This complicated the problem of inaccessible, expensive and unsafe local staples. This problem was highlighted clearly in our encounter with food hawkers at a local health centre in Amasaman (Figure 5.3). The hawkers, who had

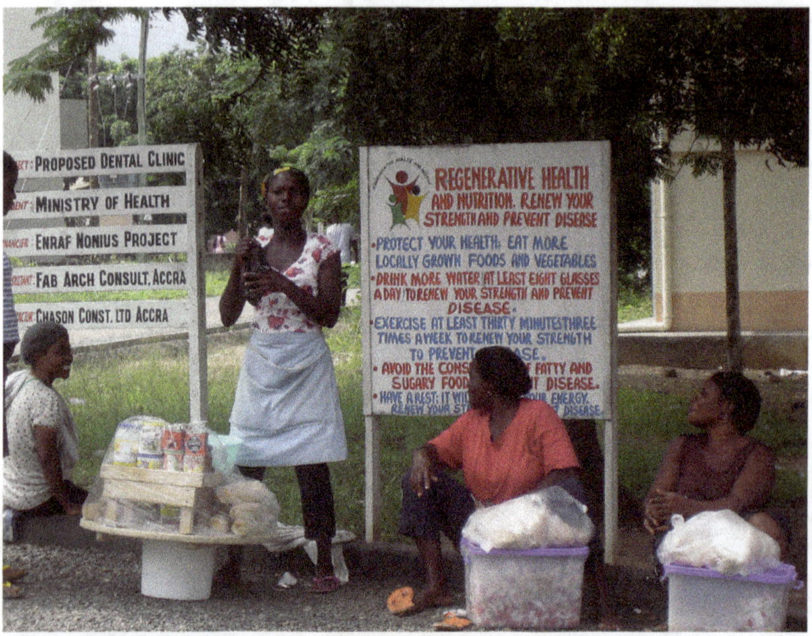
PROPOSED DENTAL CLINIC
MINISTRY OF HEALTH
ENRAF NONIUS PROJECT
FAB ARCH CONSULT. ACCRA
CHASON CONST. LTD ACCRA
REGENERATIVE HEALTH AND NUTRITION. RENEW YOUR STRENGTH AND PREVENT DISEASE
•PROTECT YOUR HEALTH: EAT MORE LOCALLY GROWN FOODS AND VEGETABLES
•DRINK MORE WATER AT LEAST EIGHT GLASSES A DAY TO RENEW YOUR STRENGTH AND PREVENT DISEASE.

Figure 5.3 Women selling ultra processed foods in front of an RHN signpost, Amasaman Health Centre.

paused to rest outside the RHN signpost, were selling the kinds of processed common daytime snacks that the RHN programme sought to prohibit – white breads baked by local bakeries, yoghurt produced by Fan Milk Limited, Ghana and margarine, mayonnaise and corned beef produced by multinational food companies.

The concerns expressed by RHN evaluation participants were not new at the time. Representations of 'toxic nutrition' had been circulating public spaces around the country and amplified in mass media headlines and narratives for years prior to the RHN programme. Across the country, and particularly in farming, fishing and mining communities, people spoke of changing diets and linked the changes to the twin challenge of toxic staples and processed foods. Lay perceptions of toxic nutrition were backed by scientific studies that reported high levels of toxic chemicals in agricultural produce, as well as rising levels of food adulteration with toxic chemicals (Amoah et al., 2006; NPAS, 2012).

The concept of 'slow violence' was advanced by American literary scholar, Rob Dixon, as 'slowly unfolding environmental catastrophes ... that are dispersed across time and space, an attritional violence that is typically not viewed as violence at all' (Nixon, 2011, cited by Davies, 2022, p.410). British geographer Thom Davies (2022) extends this concept, arguing, first, that local communities living with environmental catastrophes, see – through 'slow observations' (p.411) – live and suffer the material effects of slow violence.

> For those who live in the midst of toxic geographies and polluted landscapes, 'everyday exposure' to the accumulations of slow violence is not necessarily a 'formless threat' but can be a very real and often tangible brutality (pp.410–411).

Second, Davies argues that slow violence occurs within a broader system of structural violence and epistemic violence – these three forms of violence mutually reinforce each other. Citing Johan Galtung (1969) and Gayatri Spivak (1988), respectively, Davies defines structural violence as "suffering caused through the denial of basic needs ... when human beings are being influenced so that their actual somatic and mental realizations are below their potential" and epistemic violence as "non-formal expertise being ignored, where 'ways of knowing the world and knowing the self ... are trivialised and invalidated by Western scientists and experts'" (p.423). The intersection of structural, epistemic and slow violence was evident in the accounts of RHN participants and the broader lay and scientific accounts. In this context, it is important to note, the trivialisation and invalidation of local knowledge occurred as much through government inaction,[11] as through the influence of the country's donor partner system on policymaking.

During the evaluation phase it was clear that the slogans, 'eat more locally grown foods and vegetables'/'avoid the consumption of fatty, sugary and salty foods to prevent disease', were simplistic and problematic. Repeating the slogans did not translate into adopting corresponding RHN recipes for healthier meals. People did want to eat their local staples, especially when daily traditional meals like fufu and palmnut soup – whether cooked at home or consumed out of home – required staple food produce. They also wanted to eat more healthily by reducing foods with high fat, sugar and salt content. But the twin challenges of food toxicity and cheaper ultra-processed alternatives undermined this desire and thwarted attempts at behaviour change.

Food Is Poison: Arts and Big Food Marketing

Big Food is the label given to the "multinational food and beverage companies with huge and concentrated market power" (Stuckler and Nestle, 2012, p.1), who are blamed for the rising prevalence of nutrition-related NCDs in low- and middle-income countries like Ghana.

In Ghana, Big Food companies like Unilever and Nestle established a presence in the colonial era and have, over decades, built a formidable national infrastructure for tracking household habits and marketing their food products. National companies, like Papa Ye (a fast food restaurant) and A1 Bakery, which started local and expanded countrywide, emerged in the 1990s. In the 2000s, global fast food companies like KFC and Pizza Hut entered the local market. Big Food marketing builds on glocalisation (the intersection of global and local) principles by creating products and services for global markets that are adapted to local cultures. The adaption is done through creative methods.

Advertising copy executives for these companies understand that food, cooking, and eating are multi-sensory processes, and cuisines shape social identities. Billboards, radio and television adverts fronted by local celebrities do not only sell processed products across the major food groups – fruit, vegetables, starches, dairy and protein – that are produced to manipulate taste buds and cravings at the cellular level (Kessler, 2009;

[11] See the NPAS (2012) report.

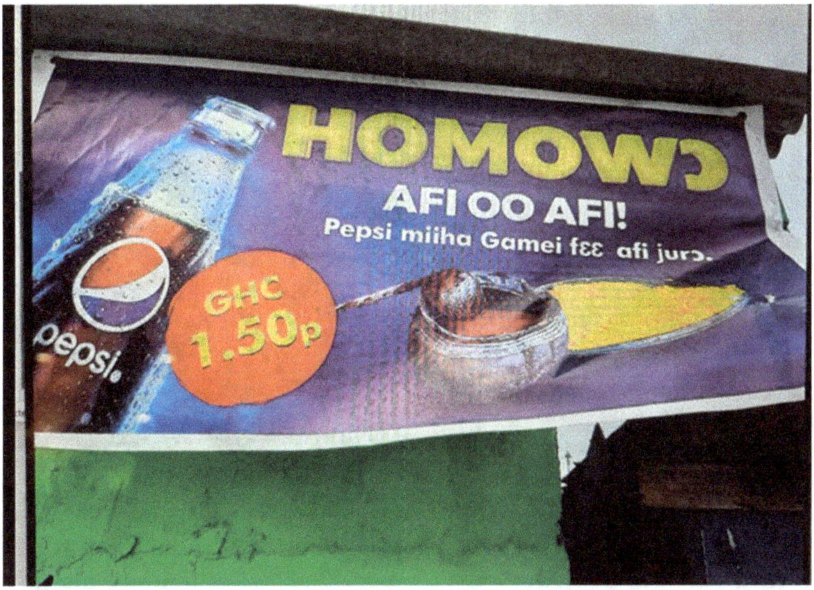

Figure 5.4 Poster of Pepsi advert during the 2022 Homowo festival, Ga Mashie. (Translation: Homowɔ Seasons Greetings! Pepsi brings to all Ga people glorious end of year greetings).

Popkin et al., 2019). They also sell lifestyle and upward mobility, enhancing the cultural imperative to look good, successful and wealthy in public – the direct opposite of ordering a meat-free meal at a chop bar, for example. To project authenticity, local languages and popular terms are used. A Pepsi poster in Ga Mashie, designed for the Homowo season, uses Ga text: *Homowɔ Afi oo Afi! Pepsi miiha Gamei fɛɛ afi jurɔ* (Homowɔ Seasons Greetings! Pepsi brings to all Ga people glorious end of year greetings)[12] (Figure 5.4). A KFC Billboard on the major George Walker Bush (GWB) Highway uses Feeli Feeli (pidgin English for seeing/feeling for yourself). The billboard, which towers over office buildings on the road, reinforces its words with a giant cut-out of chicken drumsticks cascading from a KFC bucket (Figure 5.5). An Indomie billboard, as imposing as the KFC billboard and situated on the opposite side of GWB highway, introduces a new beef flavour. Indomie, an instant noodle imported from Indonesia is an extraordinary marketing phenomenon

[12] In the poster, the Ga phonetic spelling of Homowo is used: Homowɔ. Another version is Hɔmɔwɔ.

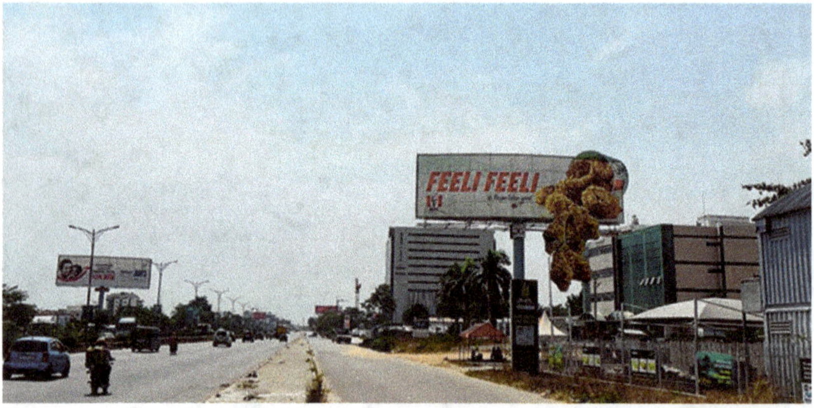

Figure 5.5 KFC billboard on George Walker Bush Highway, Accra.

in Ghana and across the African continent (Figure 5.6). Introduced to the Ghanaian market in 2006, the 'hyperpalatable' product which is packed with salt and additives was quickly absorbed into the category of national street foods and is so beloved of children and youth that Ghana's Gen Z demographic is called the Indomie Generation. Across the continent, its popularity is captured in hit songs and meals served in television dramas.[13]

Recent Big Food investments in television cookery shows hosted by local celebrities bring all the powerful arts-based marketing elements together. The award winning Edziban Food Show is broadcast on the TV3 television network. The show's host, comedian, actor and aspiring politician Kwame Dzokoto, travels round the country, visiting local chop bars and restaurants and showcasing traditional cuisines to a national audience. McBrown's Kitchen is broadcast on United Television (UTV) and hosted by the popular actor, Nana Ama McBrown. Each episode features a local or international celebrity – who talks about and cooks their favourite meal, assisted by McBrown.[14] Dzokoto's slogan – edziban ah! me

[13] Case, the popular afrobeat song released in 2018 by Nigerian singer-songwriter Teniola Apata (aka Teni) tells the story of a young couple who do not come from the extreme wealth of Nigerian billionaires, but get by on love: "Cause my papa no be Dangote, or Adeleke, but we go dey okay, yea". To underscore their working class status the song's bridge namechecks indomie, and other popular street and local foods the couple relies on for nourishment: "If nah to chop indomie, we go chop/ if nah to soak garri, we go soak/ If nah to fry akara, we go fry / If nah to soak akamu, we go soak" (see www.youtube.com/watch?v=hYx5ukr_YWw).

[14] American comedian and television host Conan O'Brien and American actor Sam Richardson appeared in McBrown's Kitchen, where they both learned to cook Jollof Rice, a dish with

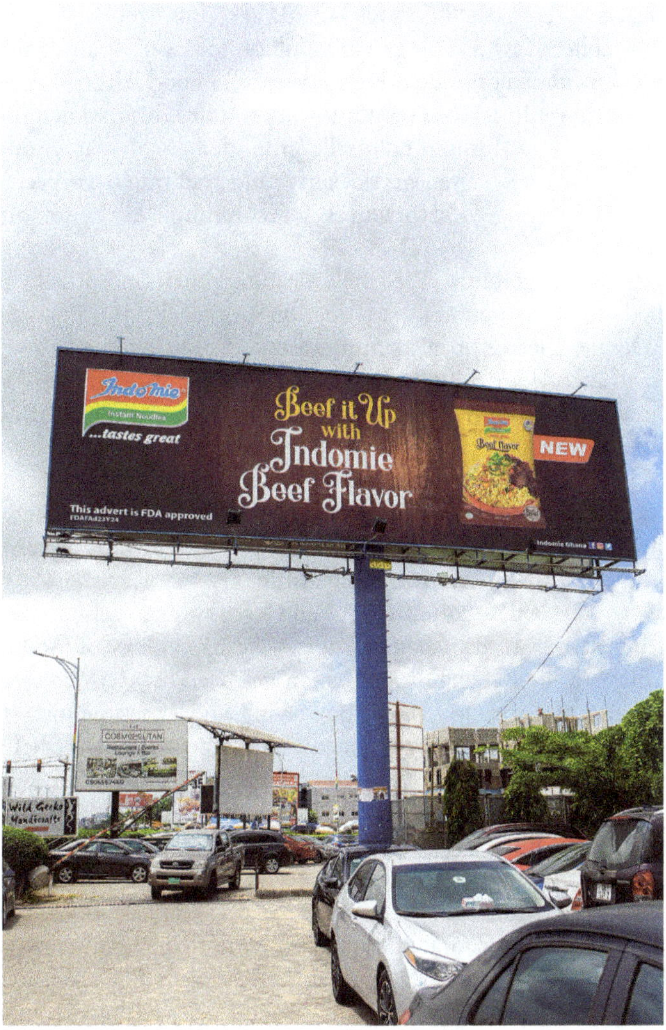

Figure 5.6 Indomie billboard on the George Walker Bush Highway, Accra.

le dzi dzi! – illustrates the way both shows emphasise the pleasures of food and eating. Both shows are sponsored by food and luxury goods companies. Both are advertised on billboards, radio, television and social

disputed West African origins, that has sparked comedic "Jollof wars" between Ghana, Nigeria and Senegal on social media (see Sloley, 2021).

media. Episodes are posted on social media accounts of TV3, UTV and of the hosts – collectively reaching over a million followers at any given time. These programmes, alongside other forms of Big Food advertising coalesce into a powerful multi-layered communication tool. This tool demonstrates that marketing food through culturally-grounded arts – that mimic taste, memory, imagination, language, sociality, and tradition – is spectacularly effective for changing food practices for communities, households and individuals.[15]

The RHN programme was well meaning but conceptually flawed. It applied an instrumental participation approach, by imposing the Edenic Divine Diet on local communities, without conducting a meaningful analysis of local food cultures or the wider food system. The art forms used for RHN messaging – which work powerfully in Big Food advertising – were superficially applied. Local collaborating experts, from the MOH, worked with the concept of 'lifestyle diseases'. This situated the risk of nutrition related chronic conditions within individual behaviour, when the 'double burden of malnutrition', then and now, is driven chiefly by commercial and environmental determinants.

Crucially, for RHN communities and communities elsewhere, these intersecting harms are also changing the social psychology of food hybridisation. Historically, Ghana's food system has been hybrid – cuisines have evolved constantly through active borrowing and experimentations with ingredients, as well as cooking and preservation techniques. Social historians observe that Ga women were selling "ready-to-eat food on the street" in the pre-colonial era, predating the "modern fast food phenomenon in America, Europe and parts of Africa" (McCann, 2010, pp.128–129). In a 1978 survey of market women in Accra, American historian Claire Robertson (1984), detailed six categories of 'ready-to-eat' foods, the preparation of which incorporated local and imported ingredients: kenkey (steamed, fermented maize dough), complete meals like fufu and soup sold in chop bars, porridge, fried snacks, baked foods and maize wine. The local fast food industry of chop bars, 'Check-Check' (fast food) joints and other forms of street food vending evolved from these Ga women pioneers and preceded the current dominance of Big Food. The Ghanaian food landscape has evolved over centuries, through glocalisation.

[15] In a move as bold as the gigantic billboard on GWB Highway, KFC has turned its marketing focus to 'catering services' and now 'caters for every occasion' including 'Weddings, Corporate events, Luncheons and Galas, Grand Openings, Funerals...' (see @KFC_Ghana posts on X).

Ghanaian geographer Joseph Mensah defines glocalisation as "the cultural interpenetration that occurs when powerful "top down" globalizing forces encounter "bottom-up processes of localization." The encounter, he argues, is dialectical: the global and local intersect in interdependent and mutually influential ways and lead to hybrid products or identities (Mensah, 2006). When Ga women reinvented new cuisines, they borrowed in deliberate ways: their curiosity led them to seek new foods and modes of cooking, and they seized opportunities afforded to coastal communities through frequent encounters with Europeans and European foods and cuisines. These glocal encounters were shaped by interconnectedness, mutual interdependence and agency – borrowings were two-way affairs, and the emerging Ga cuisines included both global and translocal elements.

Now reworking cuisines is no longer about active borrowing and experimentation. Increasingly food cultures are changing through, to resituate Mensah's (2006) argument, the imposition of 'powerful top-down globalizing forces' that stifle the agency and creativity of 'bottom-up processes of localization'. "It is even risky to eat the fresh farm produce due to the mercury deposits on the land. So now we've all turned to eating processed foods", said a participant in a photovoice study, conducted a decade after the RHN Programme, that examined perceptions of food security and nutritional health in a farming and artisanal mining community in the East Akim District (Nyantakyi-Frimpong et al., 2021, p.10). This violent interplay of expanding global forces and diminishing local choices is what nutrition interventions are up against and must contend with, whether they employ the arts or not.

CHAPTER 6

Out of Your Mind

> *"It is you people who say we are mad. I know I am sick. But mad. . .no!"* the late Lawrence Larson, a former patient at Pantang Psychiatric Hospital.

For five years, between 2003 and 2008, the Ghanaian artist and academic Bernard Akoi-Jackson volunteered as an art therapist at Pantang Psychiatric Hospital. His tenure with the hospital began when he was posted to the Occupational Therapy (OT) department as a national service person after his undergraduate degree in art at the Kwame Nkrumah University of Science and Technology (KNUST) in Kumasi.[1] There, he worked with the artist Godwin Amewu under the supervision of the head of department. The OT department provided a space for in-patients with a range of mental health conditions (and some with undiagnosed conditions)[2] to learn new skills in arts and crafts. After he completed his master's in fine arts at KNUST, he returned to the department as a postgraduate volunteer to set up an arts therapy programme. He taught painting and visual art to patients and supervised interns and national service personnel posted to the department.

Akoi-Jackson and I met in 2006 through our mutual working relationship with Ghanaian art patron Odile Tevie. He had collaborated on group art exhibitions curated by Tevie in the past. I had worked as an occasional creative writer on Tevie's arts projects. Tevie was on the verge of opening Nubuke Foundation, an arts gallery and community space situated in the East Legon suburb of Accra. Akoi-Jackson and I discovered we also had

[1] In Ghana, young people undertake a one-year national service after completing their undergraduate degrees. This scheme is coordinated by the National Service Secretariat.

[2] In a review of experiences of long-stay patients at Accra Psychiatric Hospital, hospital records showed that a sizable percentage of patients on admission and under treatment, had no formal diagnoses (de-Graft Aikins, 2015). The rates fluctuated: the percentage was 19.5 in 1960, 60.3 in 1993 and 34 in 2006.

Pantang Hospital in common. I had taught on a short course for trainee psychiatric nurses affiliated to Pantang and Ankaful Psychiatric Hospital – the second of Ghana's three psychiatric Hospitals – on a mental health capacity-building project established by the UK-based Ghanaian psychiatrist Victor Doku.[3] In the year that followed our initial meeting, I signed up to teach on a newly established Clinical Psychology Senior Clerkship – by the clinical psychologists Angela Lamensdorf Ofori-Atta and Araba Sefa-Dedeh – for medical students, with lessons held at Pantang and Accra Psychiatric Hospital (the third and Ghana's oldest psychiatric hospital). In the late 1990s I had worked with the same clinical psychologists as a graduate intern at the Accra Psychiatric Hospital, where I co-developed and led the implementation of community mental health rehabilitation projects in Accra and Kumasi.

Akoi-Jackson and I had several conversations about the value of the work he had done with patients and what we might do with the artworks they had produced over the years. A selection of the works had been included in an art exhibition curated by the French cultural organisation Alliance Française in Accra to mark a Mental Health Awareness Week. Themed 'A Different World', the exhibition showcased visual and performing arts produced in mental health institutions and 'special schools' (schools for children with various disabilities) across Ghana. Since then, the Pantang artworks had been kept in storage. Then, in 2009, Nubuke Foundation opened its doors, and Odile Tevie offered us free space and technical support to curate an exhibition.

We titled the exhibition *Out of Your Mind: Dialogues on Mental Health in Ghana*. We aimed, through the exhibition, to tell a visual story of mental illness experiences and lay perceptions of mental illness and to facilitate a dialogue with exhibition visitors. The phrase 'out of your mind' was chosen for its double meaning. On the one hand, out of your mind in colloquial English denoted 'madness' and mental distress. On the other hand, the phrase sought to examine the thoughts ('what came to mind') of exhibition visitors. We also wanted visitors to reflect on a number of questions: Was mental health merely the absence of mental illness? Why was madness (*abodam* in Twi; *sɛkɛ* in Ga) the catch-all term for mental

[3] Victor Doku established the Ghana Mental Health Educators in the Diaspora (GhMED) in the 2010s. GhMED was a network of UK-based Ghanaian mental health professionals – nurses, psychiatrists and researchers – who ran annual training sessions for mental health nurses in colleges affiliated to Pantang and Ankaful Psychiatric Hospitals and the Kintampo Rural Health Training School (now the College of Health and Wellbeing). The scheme was funded by the International Organisation for Migration (IOM) and ran for a number of years.

illnesses in Ghana? How did it feel to live with a mental illness? Who provided the best care for people living with mental illness: the psychiatrist, the herbalist, the pastor or the shrine priest? Could the creative arts help prevent or transcend mental illness?

Our joint experience working with patients and mental health professionals in psychiatric settings had introduced us to the politics of mental health care, both in terms of internal professional tensions between psychiatrists, nurses, psychologists and allied health professionals and policy inaction on funding and support for the mental health workforce. Mental health received less than 1 per cent of the country's healthcare budget, then and now.[4] The quality of services at Pantang and the other psychiatric hospitals was chronically poor as a result. For decades, hospital annual reports had detailed overcrowding, lack of medical supplies and food, and high stress levels within the workforce (Awenva et al., 2010). Therefore, we aimed to facilitate a dialogue not only on personal experiences of mental illness but also on the structural challenges in Ghanaian mental healthcare.

I will present this exhibition project and the insights it raised for applying the arts to mental health promotion and care in Ghana through a photo story and in two parts. Part One details the rationale and process of curating the exhibition. Part Two presents visitors' responses to the exhibition and two insights these revealed: the art exhibition is a viable approach for mental health promotion, and arts therapies can rehumanise the psychiatric space. In conclusion, I will reflect on what the curating process revealed about the multilayered challenges that face individuals and families affected by severe chronic mental illness and where the arts can play a role in forging more robust collaborations between psychiatric and indigenous healing systems.

Out of Your Mind: Curating the Exhibition

We curated the exhibition around five themes derived from the research evidence on mental health promotion and care needs in Ghana at the time:

(1) lay perceptions of mental illness
(2) everyday encounters with people living with mental illness

[4] In the 2023 budget statement, the government allocated a total of GH¢8,401,449,581 (equivalent to USD$763,768,143, pegged at an exchange rate of USD$1 to GH¢11) to the Ministry of Health, of which GH¢1,406,250 (equivalent to USD$127,840) was budgeted for the Mental Health Authority – a percentage of 0.016.

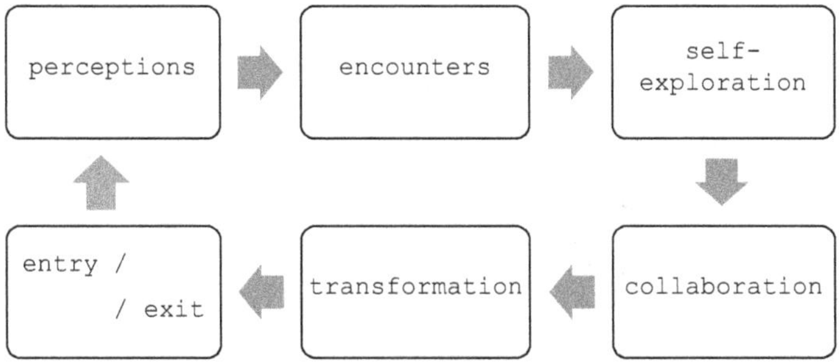

Figure 6.1 Schematic layout of the Out of Your Mind exhibition.

(3) self-exploration of lived experience in psychiatric settings
(4) collaboration through therapeutic work between patients and (art) therapists
(5) transformation of therapists' perspectives on mental illness through therapeutic work with patients

Each theme was assigned a physical space and a set of artworks and artefacts (Figure 6.1). The spaces were structured such that visitors started from outsider perspectives on mental health and illness (Perceptions) and ended with insider perspectives on lived experiences of mental illness (Transformation).

Perceptions

The Perceptions space focused on common perceptions and definitions of mental health and mental illness. This theme was captured through the commissioned paintings from seven local artists, who were asked to paint on the theme of mental health or to submit pre-existing artworks that spoke to the theme and the guiding questions. The group included established artists Kofi Setordji, Wiz Kudowor and Rikki Wemega-Kwawu, and younger artists Fatric Bewong, Dorothy Amenuke, Benedict Kojo Quaye, Patrick Tagoe-Turkson and Amenyo Dzikunu-Bansah.

The artists produced a collection of work that told similar visual stories. The submitted paintings were either abstract or figurative and rendered in bold and vivid colours. The motivation, for most artists, was to capture the way dominant lay perceptions associated mental illness with mystery and anticipated disruption and how encounters with the mentally ill evoked complicated feelings, sensations and emotions.

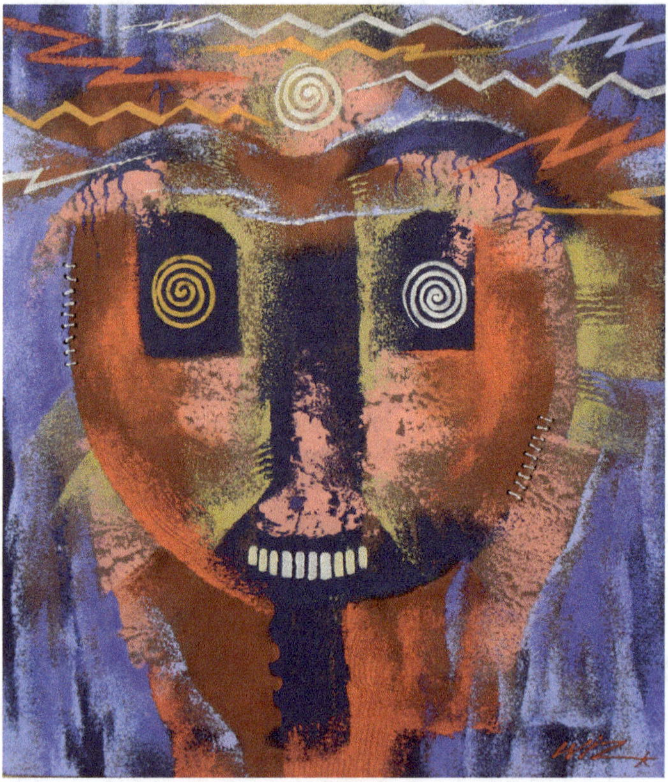

Figure 6.2 Spaced Out, painting by Wiz Kudowor.

Take, for instance, Spaced Out by Wiz Kudowor (Figure 6.2), which was painted specifically for the exhibition. The painting looked like a traditional mask used in healing rituals and festival masquerades. But instead of the inert holes that typically represent the eyes and mouth in these masks, Kudowor painted eyes that suggested dizziness or disorientation and one row of teeth, which still conjured up an image of holding emotions in check by gritting two rows of teeth. He applied vivid colours of blue, red, pink and mustard that were simultaneously complementary and distinct, and what looked like lightning striking above the head to symbolise frantic brain activity. The painting had a mesmerising quality, drawing one in and at the same time pushing one away with feelings of dread and fear. This is what I saw and felt when I first saw the painting. Kudowor explained to me that he was inspired by the general perception of mental illness as 'not being quite present or quite there in the real world' and at the same time of real internal struggles within one's headspace.

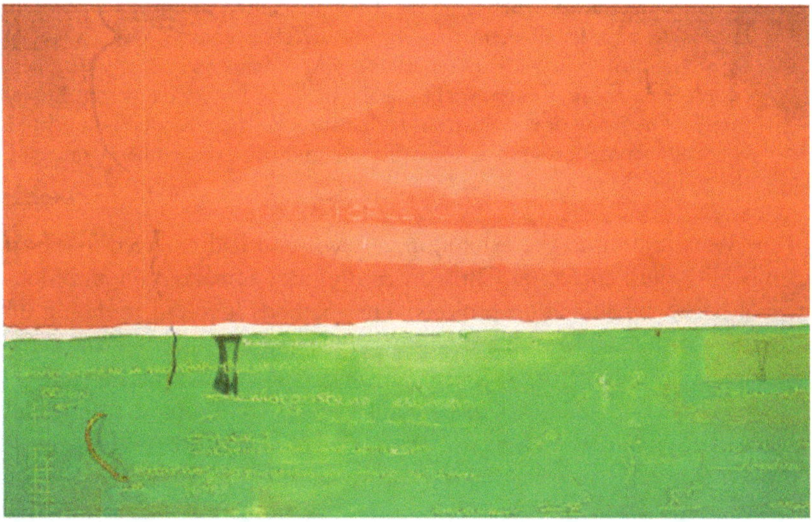

Figure 6.3 Metaphoric Boundaries, painting by Amenyo Dzikunu-Bansah.

Amenyo Dzikunu-Bansah's Metaphoric Boundaries (Figure 6.3) juxtaposed expanses of red and green separated by a white line. On both sides were eclectic letters and symbols speaking of hidden stories. Her aim, she explained, was to capture the 'metaphoric boundaries' between health (green) and illness (red) for those whose daily stressors placed their emotional state on the thin line between mental health and mental distress.

Encounters

In the *Encounters* space, we focused on two types of encounters with people living with mental illness: encounters on the streets and in indigenous healing settings. Two photographs by visual artists Riki Wemega-Kwawu and Bernard Akoi-Jackson captured encounters in the street. Encounters with homeless mentally ill individuals are commonplace on Ghanaian streets and in neighbourhoods. Every few months, there is a sensational and stigmatising headline in a Ghanaian newspaper about the rising prevalence of "lunatics" on city streets. In a quote we used in the exhibition brochure, one paper reported in March 2007 with the typical mixture of sensationalism, concern and fear:

> Lunatics are gradually besieging the Takoradi central business area with an increasing number of them roaming the streets everyday. While some of them are calm, others are hysterical and pose a danger to people, especially pedestrians. Some of them wield metals, sticks and other dangerous implements. The irony of the situation is that most of these mentally-ill people, especially women, roam the streets naked, and this is an embarrassment to the public (Marfo, 2007, p.21).

In the years leading to the exhibition, a new trend had emerged in which members of the Pentecostal Christian community embarked on ambitious mental health rehabilitation projects. The methods involved rounding up vagrants, bathing and clothing them in public, and then transporting them to rehabilitation homes or prayer camps, where they received healing prayers and exorcism. Both the mass media and religious communities imbued all vagrants with madness and, by extension, violence, or danger or evil possession. These problematic assumptions drove harmful interventions.

In the mental health literature, the "lunatics" in Ghanaian media discourse are referred to as 'vagrant psychotics'. This is a complicated category. Taha Basher and colleagues (1983, p.35) described the vagrant psychotic as:

> a person who was without permanent accommodation, employment, money or regular sources of food and who lived a socially and geographically unsettled life. He should also manifest gross abnormality of behaviour in such a way that his general conduct, emotional reactions, or cognitive functions were such that a psychotic illness could clearly be established.

Evidence over the years – from a survey conducted in Accra in the 1950s on the characteristics of vagrants to more recent official efforts to rid major cities of vagrants and beggars before important national events – suggested that not all individuals living 'socially and geographically unsettled' lives were psychotic (de-Graft Aikins, 2015).

We wanted exhibition visitors to reflect on the harmful trope of the 'lunatic/vagrant psychotic' and to see the humanity in people caught up in 'socially and geographically unsettled lives'. The photographs by Wemega-Kwawu and Akoi-Jackson brought a different perspective that facilitated such reflection. Wemega-Kwawu's photograph (Figure 6.4) captured a constellation of numbers, dates and texts inscribed on a street wall by an unnamed homeless man living in a neighbourhood in Takoradi, in the Western Region. Akoi-Jackson's photograph (Figure 6.5) captured the drawings, writings and sculptures of the late Danso, a homeless man

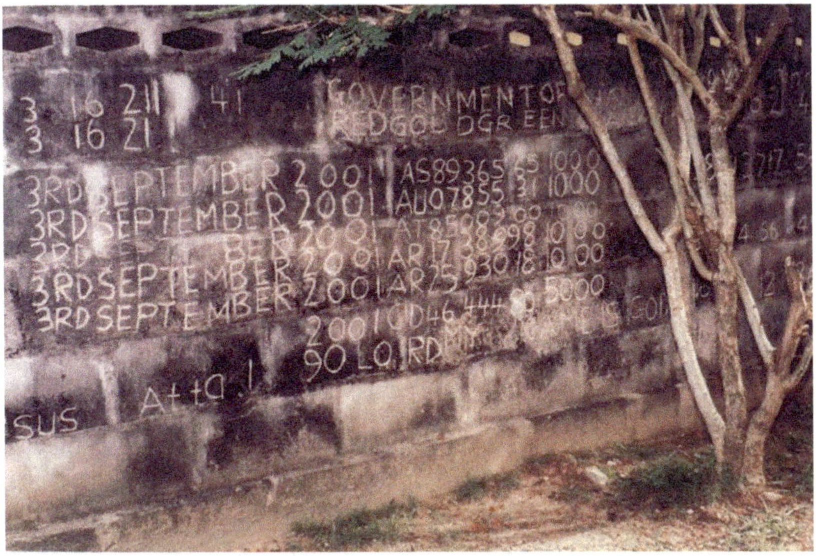

Figure 6.4 Vagrant writings on a wall, Takoradi, photograph by Rikki Wemega-Kwawu.

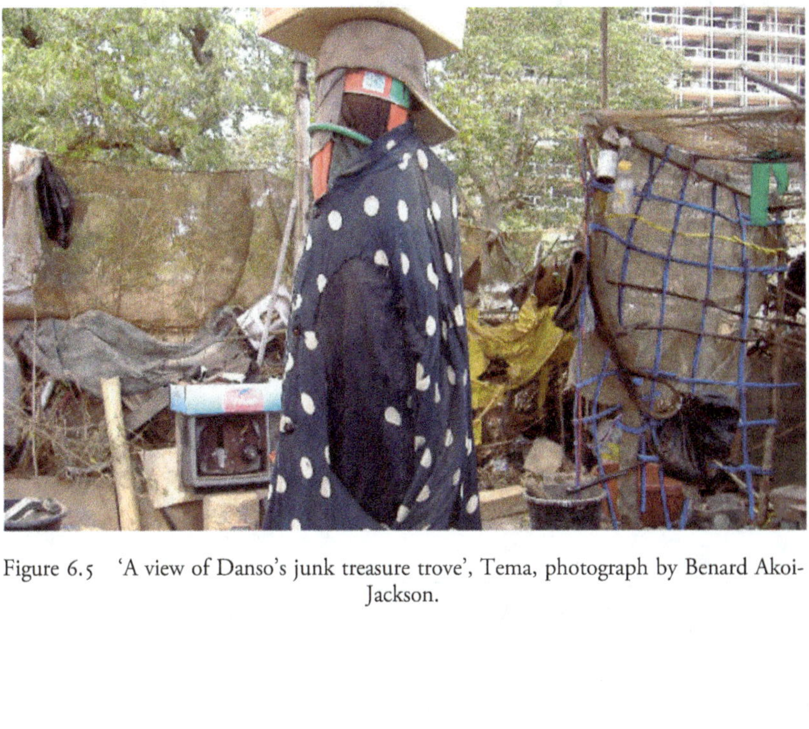

Figure 6.5 'A view of Danso's junk treasure trove', Tema, photograph by Benard Akoi-Jackson.

who had created a home on the grounds of Tema's famous but, at the time, abandoned Meridian Hotel.[5]

Both artists believed that the repetition of form and content in the material productions of the homeless men spoke of important events and concerns in their past. The photographs provided a glimpse of their interior lives by capturing their creative expressions under precarious living conditions.

Ursula Read, a British anthropologist and former occupational therapist, provided photographs that focused on encounters in indigenous healing settings. The photographs were taken as part of her doctoral ethnographic research with individuals and families affected by chronic mental illness in Kintampo (Read et al., 2009). About 70 per cent of Ghana's population is rural and is underserved by mental health services. The three psychiatric hospitals are located in cities in the country's south, and community mental health services are understaffed and underfunded. Therefore, the challenges faced by rural and northern families caring for mentally ill relatives are particularly harrowing. But Read's visual anthropological story also applied to family experiences of mental illness across the country, then and now.

Many seriously mentally ill individuals are cared for predominantly within family settings. Serious mental health conditions are often attributed to spiritual factors. Therefore, treatment choices begin in spaces of spiritual healing. Read's photographs captured healing journeys in traditional shrines, prayer camps (Figure 6.6) and Pentecostal churches (Figure 6.7). Within these healing spheres, mental illness is often believed to be the product of evil or spirit possession. Exorcism is conducted through prayer, fasting and beating spirits out of the possessed (Figure 6.7). Another key aspect of treatment in all these institutions is restraint. At prayer camps and traditional shrines, patients are chained to trees, rocks, logs, furniture and other solid contraptions to prevent them from harming themselves or others (Figure 6.6). They are often left outside at all hours and under all weather conditions. In the family settings Read observed, individuals whose symptoms had abated or whose behaviours did not pose a threat to themselves or family members were allowed to engage with the community outside their home. For one family, the freedom came with draconian conditions – a heavy log tied to their relative's left foot to prevent him from straying too far from home (Figure 6.8).

[5] Meridian Hotel was so popular in the 1970s that it was immortalised in the Ga highlife song Meridian by the Wulomei band.

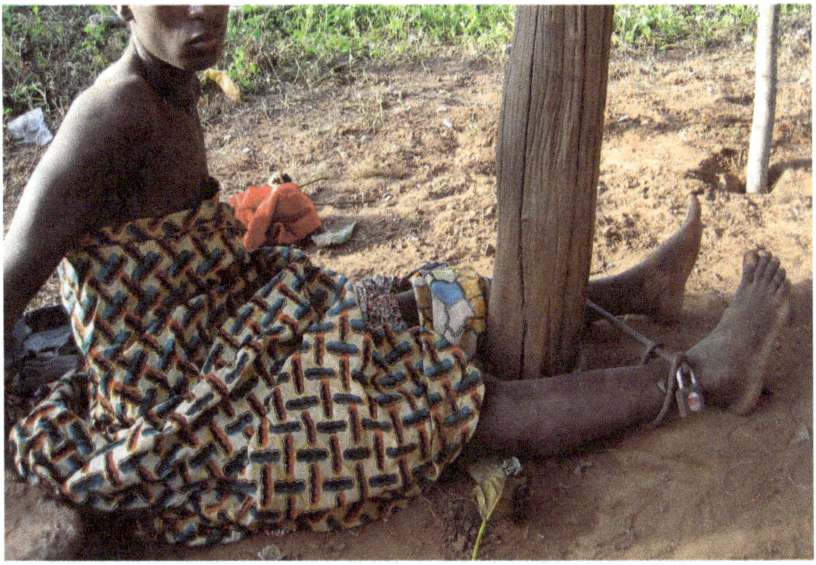

Figure 6.6 Woman in a prayer camp, Kintampo, photograph by Ursula Read.

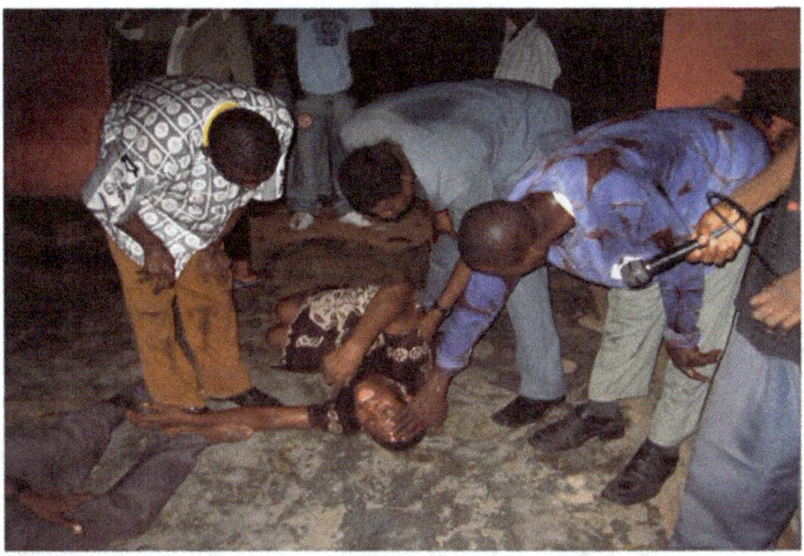

Figure 6.7 Casting out evil spirits at a Pentecostal church, Kintampo, photograph by Ursula Read.

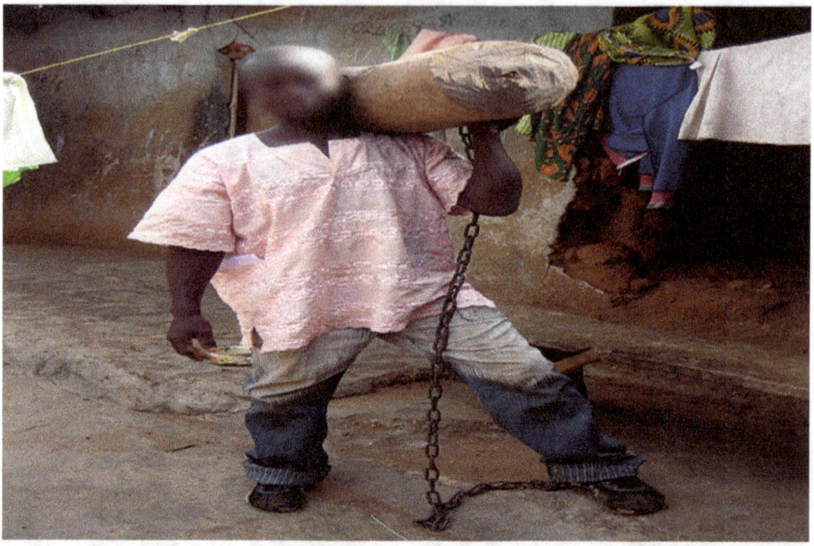

Figure 6.8 Man with a log, Kintampo, photograph by Ursula Read.

Self-Exploration

The *Self-Exploration* space focused on lived experiences of mental illness in psychiatric settings. Akoi-Jackson worked with long-stay patients. This is a category of patients – in Pantang Hospital and the other two psychiatric hospitals – who were institutionalised, having spent several years in one ward or across several wards. Some patients within this category experienced a revolving door process, which involved transitions between discharge and readmission over several years.

A group of eight patients – six men and two women – diagnosed with depression, substance abuse disorders and schizophrenia, worked with Bernard Akoi-Jackson between 2004 and 2008. They switched between the art therapy he provided and occupational therapy provided by the OT staff. During art therapy sessions they produced sketches, colourings on paper, paintings on canvas and clay objects. During occupational therapy sessions, they produced craftwork including baskets, wood products, cushions and stuffed objects.

Akoi-Jackson and his group discussed the inspiration behind their creative work. For some individuals, the artistic products captured emotions of the past, of a given day, or of an imagined future, typically post-discharge. For others, their creative expression described their identities: who they were before illness struck, who they were in relation to

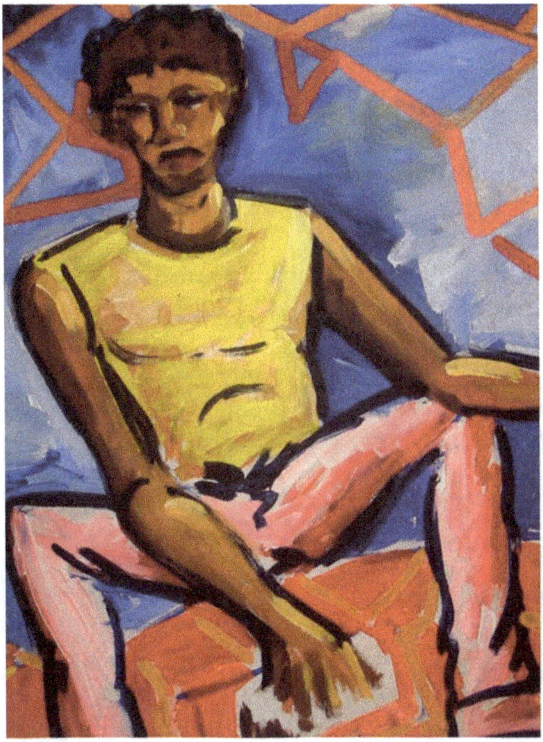

Figure 6.9 Shoeshine Boy, painting by Kwame.

significant others and their institutional caregivers, and who they hoped to become after discharge.

The paintings, crafts and objects produced by individual patients were exhibited in the Self-exploration space. One long-stay patient, Kwame,[6] produced a series of paintings during Akoi-Jackson's tenure. His paintings focused on two major themes that mattered to him: faith and livelihood. One of the paintings, titled Shoeshine Boy (Figure 6.9), captured his concern for young Ghanaian men who worked precarious jobs on the streets.

Collaboration

Collaboration focused on the collaborative processes between therapist and client. Effective therapy aims for collaborative empiricism. This is the

[6] Name has been changed to protect his identity.

process through which a therapist and their client work together to construct meanings about the illness experience and to develop practical approaches for recovery and flourishing (Overholser, 2011). Typically used in cognitive behavioural therapy (CBT), where the relationship is between a patient and therapist and the focus is on deconstructing disordered thinking and debilitating beliefs, the core principle of co-constructing meaning and action works in group-based therapies also. At the time of the exhibition, group therapy was offered to individuals addicted to alcohol and narcotic drugs in Ghana but remained unexplored for other conditions (Read and Doku, 2012). Patients worked in groups with

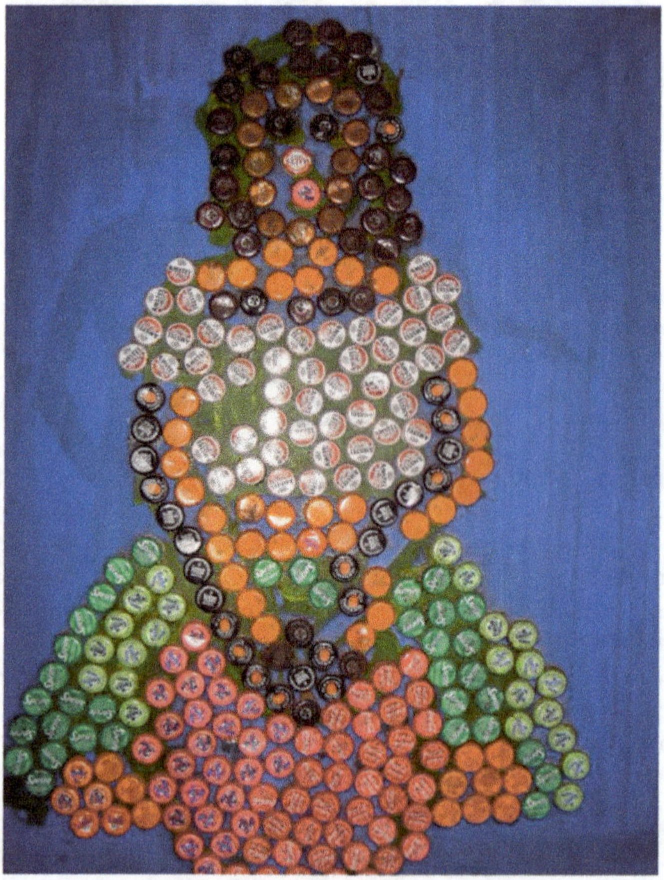

Figure 6.10 Woman in Dress, painting by Yaganoma Baatoulkuu and a group of patients.

Bernard Akoi-Jackson, Godwin Amewu and art interns like Yaganoma Baatuolkuu at different periods between 2003 and 2008. These group sessions produced mixed media paintings, prints made from natural materials such as leaves and tree barks, clay objects and other artefacts. Through the collaborative process, a range of themes were explored, including experiencing and managing mental and emotional flux at home and in the psychiatric wards. *Woman in Dress* (Figure 6.10) was a mixed media painting produced by Yaganoma Baatuolkuu and patients with paint and bottle tops. The painting focused on women's mental health and aimed to capture beauty, poise and resilience in the face of mental distress.

Transformation

The Transformation space examined the transformative experience of working with psychiatric patients. Ursula Read observed in the exhibition brochure:

> Working with people in mental distress makes you a witness to human sensitivity, to mistakes and failures, disappointments and sadness. At the same time you see amazing human strength, resilience and creativity, as people put their lives back together, rebuild relationships, and cope with challenges and tragedies.

Akoi-Jackson produced several paintings that were inspired by the patients he worked with over the years. Each interpretative painting was informed by observing the spontaneous process through which a patient produced their piece of art, followed by conversations with the patient about the content and meaning of the artistic product. In one conversation on representations of madness with Lawrence Larson, a patient he had worked with for years, Akoi-Jackson asked Larson: So can you tell a 'madman' when you see one? Lawson responded:

> I cannot undermine the integrity of a fellow man. It is you people who say we are mad. I know I am sick. But mad [. . .] no!

Some of the paintings were re-interpretations of patients' work. Others were visual representations of themes that emerged during conversations with patients, such as the conversation with Larson (Figure 6.11). Akoi-Jackson's therapeutic work with patients transformed him beyond experimentation with painting media and styles. The experience

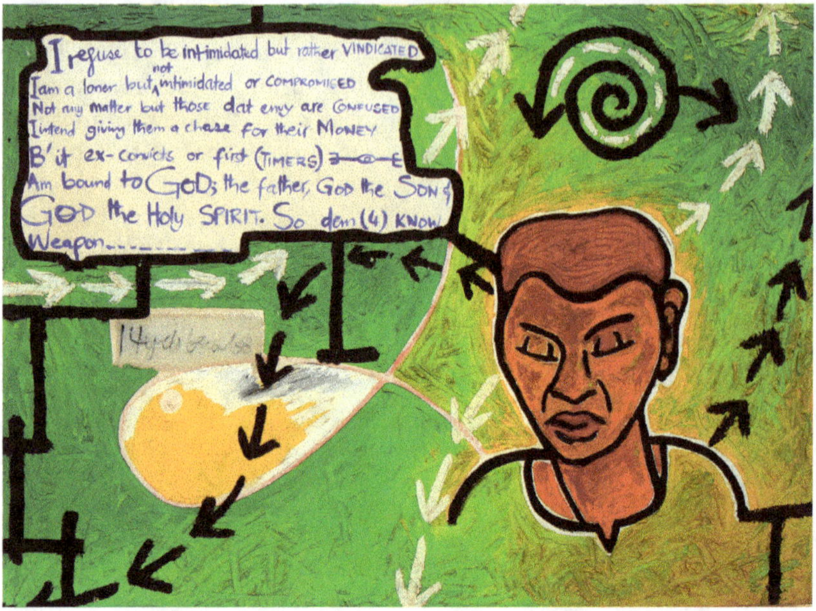
I refuse to be intimidated but rather VINDICATED
I am a loner but not intimidated or COMPROMISED
Not my matter but those dat envy are CONFUSED
I intend giving them a chase for their MONEY
B' it ex-convicts or first (TIMERS)
Am bound to GOD; the father, GOD the SON &
GOD the Holy SPIRIT. So dem (4) KNOW
Weapon.........

Figure 6.11 For Larson, painting by Bernard Akoi-Jackson.

inspired him to engage in mental health advocacy. He introduced additional actors to expand the artistic experiences of patients at Pantang Hospital, such as Performing Arts students from the University of Ghana, who engaged staff and patients in music, drama and dance sessions. He also raised funding from local charitable organisations to support refurbishments at the OT department.

"A Very Powerful Exhibition": Visitors' Responses

The exhibition opened on 15 February 2009 at the Nubuke Foundation to over one hundred visitors from the mental health, research and arts communities and media. Odile Tevie and the Polish medical director of Pantang Hospital, Dr Anna Puklo-Dzadey, introduced the event. Osei Kwame Korankye, a veteran *seprewa* (a traditional Akan harp-lute) musician, was commissioned to perform a bespoke praise song recital for the event. Sitting in the reception area, where visitors entered and exited, he performed the recital at regular intervals, providing a musical backdrop to the exhibition experience.

The exhibition showed for one week, during which more visitors attended, including students, nurses and patients from Pantang Psychiatric Hospital. We conducted exit interviews with the exhibition visitors on the opening day and collated written reviews in a visitors' book. Exit interviews were also conducted with nurses and patients who visited during the week. The exhibition was featured on a *BBC Focus on Africa* radio programme, on Ghana Television(GTV) and in the *Daily Graphic*. The data and team reflections of the exhibition process yielded two major insights: first, the art exhibition was a viable method of mental health promotion; second, art therapies could 'rehumanise' the psychiatric space.

The majority of exit interviewees described the visual stories of lived experiences of mental illness as compelling and thought-provoking. Visitors reported an emotional connection with artwork produced by patients and the anthropological photographs and a selection of the artists' paintings. Wiz Kudowor's Spaced Out (Figure 6.2) and Ursula Read's anthropological photographs (Figures 6.6–6.8) were singled out as impactful exhibits.

> 'Spaced Out' touched me really well [. . .] Many of us are in that situation, trying to find our way out.

Most visitors had little knowledge of the scale and impact of mental health problems in Ghana and, especially, of rural experiences. The stories presented through the exhibits, and the research evidence and statistics provided in the exhibition brochure, were described as educational.

> The issue of chaining was very surprising and something I was not aware of.

Visitors provided feedback on the value of the art exhibition as a vehicle for mental health promotion. Some commented on the value of collecting art produced by psychiatric patients and establishing a regular space for showing this kind of art.

> looking at the impressions mental patients can put on paper, I think it is right that they are not ignored, but we work with them to speed up their recoveries

> a very powerful exhibition – seeing the sounds of unheard voices; and insight into turmoil, suffering but with the hope of being able to communicate. This could be a regular exhibition with a growing collection of this type of art

Curating art produced by patients and artists generated a nuanced visual story of mental illness that took on lived experiences and social representations. Psychiatric patients are typically locked away, unseen by extended family and outsiders. Having their creative work shown in public was a powerful way of bringing their lives to the fore and showing that the ability to imagine, create and produce did not diminish when one lived with a mental illness, even within the confines of a psychiatric hospital.

The exhibition brought together local artists who painted on the theme for the first time or reconceptualised existing artworks through the theme of mental health and mental illness. The process of curating, bringing the artworks to the exhibition space and having conversations during the preparation process provided insights into how this group of creatives absorbed social representations of mental illness circulating in public and also how future collaborations – such as group exhibitions on mental health and other health conditions – could be organised.

Exit interviews with nurses and patients who visited the exhibition during the week, and with a former patient who participated in Akoi-Jackson's art therapy sessions, suggested the art therapy sessions had a twofold impact. The creative process helped patients to deal with the stress of ward experiences, and the nurses who assisted in sessions reported similar stress-reduction benefits for themselves. This dual impact improved the quality of relationships between patients and nurses and had the potential to improve the quality of life in the hospital. Mental healthcare professionals are poorly paid, work under stressful conditions and, for those who work in psychiatric hospitals, experience courtesy stigma (Awenva et al., 2010). These dynamics have been associated with poor quality care of patients, burnout among mental healthcare professionals and a high attrition rate within segments of the profession. The finding that arts-based interventions could improve the well-being of participating ward nurses offered a practical approach – albeit one that required art therapists and funding – to rehumanise everyday relationships between patients and healthcare professionals.

Arts and Pluralistic Mental Healing

Out of Your Mind used arts to tell the story of lived experiences of mental illness in one psychiatric institution. But the process of curating the exhibition revealed an underlying story of structural barriers to mental healthcare in Ghana and of an uneasy co-existence between psychiatric and indigenous healing services. Since Accra Psychiatric Hospital was opened in 1906, official mental healthcare has been consistently under-resourced and under-funded. A mental health law passed over a century later, in 2012, placed emphasis on community-based mental healthcare, but the number of community mental health nurses is low and those at post are not adequately equipped to provide services, such as having transport to pay house calls. The mental health budget has remained at less than one per cent of the national health budget for decades. Mental health services are therefore largely run on charity. Small groups from churches, businesses and schools and wealthy individuals provide ad hoc support to the frequently needy psychiatric hospitals, such as food supplies and financial donations. Akoi-Jackson's advocacy efforts during his tenure at Pantang fall under this category. Larger national-level advocacy organisations like Basic Needs and the Mental Health Society of Ghana work alongside the Mental Health Authority – the statutory body that sets the guidelines for and evaluates services – to address the financial and human resource challenges that cripple institutional and community-based care.

Due to these chronic systemic challenges, periodic attempts have been made to forge collaborations between psychiatric services, shrines and prayer camps. In the 1960s, a short-lived pilot project explored the establishment of a village settlement for discharged patients, drawing on the model of residential shrine-based healing (Barnor, 2001). More recently, a team of psychiatrists and clinical psychologists piloted a randomised control trial of faith and pharmacological treatment in prayer camps (Ofori-Atta et al., 2018). These small-scale projects have typically framed the collaborations through a lens of biomedical superiority and ethnomedical inferiority, when in reality each system is fallible and often in similar ways. Restraint, for example, is used across the systems: while shrines and prayer camps restrain physically, psychiatric hospitals immobilise patients through psychotropic medication. Patients who healer-shop across these major systems express dissatisfaction with treatment approaches, and there are frequent attempts by some patients to escape.

A recent award-winning film, *Nkabom: a little medicine, a little prayer*, directed by visual anthropologist Erminia Colucci, offers new insights.[7] Developed through a funded interdisciplinary project and building on community relationships established through Ursula Read's doctoral study, the film followed community mental health nurses in Nkoranza and Kintampo as they sought to build collaborative working relationships with prayer camp leaders and shrine priests. Visual vignettes of lived experiences in these spaces formed the core of the film. Patients and caregivers who had healer-shopped across systems for years offered insights into indigenous healing practices that gave them psychological and

[7] The film is available on YouTube at www.youtube.com/watch?v=b5dd_oNrRaA (last accessed 15 March 2024).

spiritual relief, such as singing and dancing – alone or in groups – and experiencing the laying on of hands.[8]

The clinical benefits of indigenous psychotherapy techniques – for example, the use of 'ritual baths' in Ga shrine treatment repertoires (Mullings, 1984, see Chapter 2) or body art and dance in Ewe shrines (Adjei, 2020) – have not been systematically studied by local mental health researchers. But these 'sensory' and 'embodied' techniques are reported in the global mental health literature to reduce distress and minimise re-traumatisation in psychiatric wards (Scanlan and Novak, 2015). In some post-conflict community settings, where chronic mental health problems are rooted in collective trauma, local arts traditions have been incorporated into mental health interventions. In Rwanda, American art therapist Valerie Chu (2010) facilitated group therapy sessions with eight young adult survivors of the 1994 genocide, following five summers of therapeutic engagement with their broader community. The sessions involved the creation of 'self-boxes': plain cardboard boxes that each young person – given "scraps of local fabric, crayons, markers, paper, scissors, glue, and magazine images" (p.6) – decorated with images and texts and filled with objects of personal meaning. The box represented a vessel of storage: "as a container [it] connected with the larger, important role of containers within Rwandan culture" (Chu, 2020 p.6), such as baskets. Chu observed that 'open displays of personal emotion' were not encouraged in Rwandan culture – this cultural imperative was captured in proverbs such as "the tears of a man flow within" (p.6). Therefore, the box was also used as a metaphor for the private release of complicated emotions associated with trauma. By choosing an art method that was culturally grounded, participants were guided to explore their identities and express their emotions in ways that were simultaneously culturally appropriate and self-affirming. Chu reported that the sessions catalysed "expression, healing, and reconnection with the self" thereby fostering post-traumatic growth (p.4).

Mental health policy in Ghana is largely rhetorical. The reality, therefore, is that people living with chronic mental illness will be caught within the revolving door of pluralistic mental healing. Collaborative treatments that blend the pharmacological, spiritual and creative in culturally grounded ways that promote growth and independence offer the chance of a better quality of life with chronic mental illness.

[8] "The ritual act in which a priest places one or both hands palms down on the top of another person's head, usually while saying a prayer or blessing" (Encyclopaedia Britannica, www.britannica.com/topic/imposition-of-hands).

CHAPTER 7

We Cannot Eat Stories

> "Kɛji wɔtã adesai lɛ, kɛkɛ lɛ mɛni? Adesai lɛ amɛjeee niyenii ni wɔbaaye"/"We tell the stories and then what? We cannot eat stories".
>
> Nii Sampa Kojo, a member of Jamestown Health Club.

In 2019, the NCD Alliance – the global civil society network dedicated to noncommunicable diseases (NCD) advocacy – developed a storytelling project called *Our Views, Our Voices.* The project was described as part of a global initiative to "enable individuals living with NCDs to share their views to take action and drive change".[1] They organised training workshops on NCD storytelling in a number of countries in partnership with national NCD Alliances, including Ghana NCD Alliance (hereafter GhNCDA). GhNCDA published a local advert on Twitter (now X), calling for English speakers (only) to apply for limited spaces for training. My research team applied to have two members of Jamestown Health Club – Nii Sampa Kojo and Rosemond Aku Allotey – participate in the training.[2] At our next monthly meeting we asked for a brief report. Nii Sampa said sarcastically, in Ga, and to laughter within the group: "[W]e tell the stories and then what? We cannot eat stories." Nii Sampa's critique revealed the double-edged nature of storytelling as an advocacy method in global health.

In narrative health, studies explore how health attitudes and health behaviour can be changed through storytelling and story listening. A variety of methods have been used, including patient testimonials, story-writing competitions, short films and long-running soap operas (Bunn et al., 2020; Frank et al., 2015; Pallai and Tran, 2019; Sonke and Pesata, 2015).

[1] Visit: https://ncdalliance.org.

[2] Nii Sampa Kojo and Rosemond Aku Allotey granted permission for their names to be used in this chapter. Nii Sampa and Sister Aku, as they are called by club members, represent the club at national NCD-related events organised by GhNCDA and other organisations.

When audiences encounter stories from individuals with lived experience of illness, through patient testimonials, or from well-crafted fictionalised versions of common experiences, through film or soap operas, they are transported into a narrative world, through 'a distinct mental process' which involves "a convergence of attention, imagery, and feelings" (Frank et al., 2015, p.155). If the characters in the stories are sympathetic and recognisable, audiences can "assume the identity, goals, and perspective of a character" through an imaginative process (Frank et al., 2015, p.156). The act of telling stories also has benefits. It "allows the storyteller to connect their physical health to their mental, social, religious, and other realms of health" (Pallai and Tran, 2019, p.2). This holistic process might lead, in some instances, to self-empowerment and self-transformation (Krause, 2003; Nguyen, 2010). When storytelling interventions are longitudinal, such as when health storylines are woven into long-running soap operas, these psychological processes can translate not only to intentions to change health behaviours but also to measurable behavioural change (Frank et al., 2015).

However, storytelling, like all arts-based health methods, has limitations. In narrative health, critiques have centred on how stories are structured, who tells the story, who listens to the story and who benefits from the story (Frank et al., 2015; Pallai and Tran, 2019). Firstly, not all stories can be told in entirety and publicly. Stigmatised health conditions can be challenging to describe through either true or fictional stories, as HIV and mental health stories have shown (Bunn et al., 2020; Costa et al., 2012). Secondly, if storylines and characters do not reflect the social and cultural realities or moral codes of the intended audience, listeners are unlikely to engage and adapt the messaging. Critics of storytelling in global health focus on the politics of how particular stories are chosen for targeted communities with health needs and the purposes these stories serve for various actors (Tyler and Slater, 2018).

When the NCD Alliance *Our Views, Our Voices* project (hereafter the OVOV project) came to Accra, there had been at least twenty years of NCD advocacy by patient support groups. Stories shared by these groups had contributed to shifting perceptions and understandings of common chronic conditions like diabetes, hypertension and stroke. Applying a narrative health framework, I will describe the encounter between the OVOV project and the local patient support movement, focusing on the method of storytelling used by both sets of actors: the patient testimonial. For support groups, the patient testimonial has been used in its simple form: real life stories of lived experiences of chronic illness. The NCD

Alliance applied a stylised version, which Vinh-Kim Nguyen (2010) refers to as a 'confessional technology'. Drawing on the ideas of French philosopher Michel Foucault (1988), Nguyen defined confessional technologies as "technologies of the self": "a ritual of discourse" and "practices that permit individuals to effect by their own means or with the help of others a certain number of operations on their own bodies, thoughts, conduct and way of being [...] to transform the self" for personal gain such as happiness and wisdom (p.39). But depending on the situational context – such as the Christian confession which shaped Foucault's ideas – "confessional technologies [are] also political technologies, reproducing forms of power between individuals and agencies that require the confession" (p.39). I will examine the extent to which patient testimonials and confessional technologies intersect – positively or negatively – with the political technologies of the NCD Alliance and government actors. I will then reflect on the scope and limits of storytelling as a means for 'taking action and driving change' for NCD prevention and control in Ghana.

'Our Views, Our Voices'?

In *The Republic of Therapy: Triage and Sovereignty in West Africa's Time of AIDS*, Vinh-Kim Nguyen (2010) presents a powerful example of the double-edged nature of storytelling during the early decades of the HIV/AIDS pandemic. As HIV prevalence grew across the African continent and government responses remained static, the patient testimonial became central to AIDS advocacy. Courageous individuals who spoke up about their lived experiences were co-opted into 'the global AIDS industry' of testimonials and support groups. This industry was powered by 'confessional technologies'. HIV confessional technologies were taught in workshops, which were designed through advocacy activities initiated by the gay community in California in the first decade of the HIV/AIDS pandemic. These workshops became the dominant intervention in African countries, including in Côte d'Ivoire and Burkina Faso, where Nguyen carried out his ethnographic work. At the workshops, participants were taught how to build trust, role-play, "to master the arts of asking, telling, listening" (p.8) and the deployment of relational emotions, such as empathy, to forge 'caring relationships' and elicit stories of lived experiences.

The workshops encountered 'technical difficulties'. In one workshop Nguyen observed, some aspects of the technology were accepted, others challenged. For example, participants learned listening skills that helped them manage interpersonal relationships, and some participants brought their personal struggles into role-play in order to get free advice. But once the techniques entered the outside world, they "collided with a dense local economy of ideas and practices of the self that interfered with their seamless transfer from North to South" (p.49). Ideas that did not take on psychosocial struggles around disclosure, urgent medical and medicine needs, and the fragility of relationships in the context of HIV/AIDS were not workable. For many, telling stories or eliciting the stories of others through their newly acquired skills did not address the material or medical impact of living with HIV or having HIV-related care responsibilities: "good deeds were measured in terms of relief from symptoms, not in stories told" (p.52).

The NCD Alliance storytelling project adopted the same approach as the HIV workshops. At a fundamental branding level, when the Alliance became an official umbrella organisation of the Union for International Cancer Control (UICC), World Heart Federation (WHF), International Union of TB and Lung Disease and International Diabetes Federation (IDF) in 2017, the focal chronic conditions of these long-standing organisations were subsumed under the NCD label. Following PLWHAs, the acronym describing people living with HIV/AIDS, people with cancers, heart disease, chronic respiratory conditions and diabetes – conditions that had distinct clinical causes, profiles and prognoses – became PLWNCDs: 'people living with NCDs'. If the rebranding was a mouthful in English, it created even more linguistic confusion among people for whom English was not the primary language. Diabetes, heart disease and cancers had local language versions, but how did one say and explain PLWNCDs in Fante, Ga, Ewe or Dagbani? The storytelling project involved training local collaborators, GhNCDA staff, in a standardised storytelling method, which they had to impart to 'PLWNCDs'. Workshops – the medium of instruction – were convened in three cities: Accra, Kumasi and Tamale. The language of instruction was English.

The NCD workshops, like the HIV precursors, encountered 'technical difficulties'. Labram Musah, National Coordinator of GhNCDA, noted that GhNCDA staff struggled to recruit participants for the storytelling training sessions beyond individuals living with "already known conditions like diabetes and hypertension".[3] Individuals living with stigmatised conditions, like cancers, were not willing to tell their stories. Four stories eventually made it to the NCD Alliance website and social media platforms.

[3] Interview with Labram Musah, April 2023.

Christopher Agbeba shared his personal story of living with hereditary motor sensory neuropathy.[4] Katherine Berkoh shared her story of living with endometriosis and advocating for women ('endo warriors') with the condition.[5] Ama Quainoo's story focused on living with sickle-cell disease.[6] Vivian Gyasi Sarfo told her story of living with breast cancer and hypertension.[7] Each life story was unique and shed light on the medical profiles and psychosocial impact of distinct chronic conditions. But some themes cut across the four stories, including late diagnoses, prohibitive cost of specialist treatments and medicines, anticipated and lived stigma, healer-shopping, and the urgent need for improved NCD care.

These personal stories were designed for personal empowerment as well as for social and health systems change in local country contexts.[8] By their own accounts, sharing personal stories allowed Agbeba, Berkoh, Quainoo and Sarfo to take charge of their lives and capabilities as NCD advocates. "Everything becomes a little different as soon as it is spoken out" Ama Quainoo observed. However, 'driving change' for NCD control and prevention in Ghana was a more complicated task, as we will see when we place the personal story within the context of the patient support group movement.

The Story of ShareCare Ghana

ShareCare Ghana (hereafter SCG) was established by former journalist Nana Yaa Agyeman (NYA) in 2007 to address the needs of individuals living with autoimmune and neurological conditions.[9] A few years prior, she had been diagnosed with multiple sclerosis after an eight-year search for a medical diagnosis.

> It was in 2003 that I was diagnosed with multiple sclerosis. But my condition started in 1995. I was working as a journalist for a number of years and at the time I got ill, I was just about to join a new radio station.

4 Visit: www.ourviewsourvoices.org/ncd-diaries/equity-and-uhc/christopher-agbeba.

5 Visit: www.ourviewsourvoices.org/ncd-diaries/universal-health-coverage/katherine-berkoh.

6 Visit: www.ourviewsourvoices.org/ncd-diaries/the-experience-of-living-with-multiple-chronic-conditions/ama-quainoo.

7 Visit: www.ourviewsourvoices.org/ncd-diaries/the-experience-of-living-with-multiple-chronic-conditions/vivian-gyasi-sarfo.

8 Other diary podcasts and written diaries showcase personal stories from twenty-four countries including, ten African countries: Cameroon, Ghana, Malawi, Nigeria, Rwanda, Sierra Leone, Tanzania, Togo, Uganda and Zambia.

9 This story is based on interviews conducted with Nana Yaa Agyeman in 2021 and with Christopher Agbeba in 2021 and 2023. Audio and transcripts of the 2021 interviews are available at www.chronicitycareafrica.com. Nana Yaa Agyeman passed away in August 2022. Her family granted permission in August 2023 for the interviews to be re-used in this chapter.

> I just started getting sick, moving from hospital to hospital not knowing what was going on. Until finally I was almost paralyzed from the leg down. That was really the beginning of the journey, 25 years ago.

She and her family felt others had to be going through a similar experience and might need information and support:

> So we put the message out, and the word that came to mind is to share what I am going through. That was the beginning of ShareCare, which later became ShareCare Ghana.

Christopher Agbeba (CA) recalls first seeing Nana Yaa Agyeman on the television chat show KSM in 2007:[10]

> Immediately I saw her interview, and the things she was talking about, I realised that okay, this condition that she's talking about, has some similarities to what I'm currently experiencing. So, they used to meet at a place in the Airport area [*a wealthy suburb of Accra*] and I met them.

He was in senior high school then and had not yet received his diagnosis. It took nine years of doctor-shopping at various clinics and the Korle-Bu Teaching Hospital, interspersed with visits to pastors and prayer camps, to get the diagnosis of hereditary motor sensory neuropathy (also known as Charcot-Marie-Tooth disease). Christopher's father had the same condition, but his symptoms had not been fully understood by the family.

> My dad had it. [But] they didn't seek for medical attention. They didn't have a medical understanding to what was going on. So, growing up, I thought my dad had an accident. Then I started experiencing the symptoms in 2006, 2007. And then that was when I started asking questions, I was getting answers. I realized that, okay, this was much deeper than I thought it was.

ShareCare Ghana launched formally in June 2008 at the Ghana College of Physicians and Surgeons, Accra, with support from medical and research groups. Christopher Agbeba took on the role of SCG's Advocacy Manager. The group joined the Ghana Federation of Disability Organisations (GFD), an umbrella organisation for nine organisations, which had been formed after years of multi-stakeholder lobbying and consultations. SCG and the Mental Health Society of Ghana (MEHSOG) were the only members that dealt specifically with chronic diseases. The other member organisations focused on physical, cognitive and 'psychosocial'

[10] The *KSM Show* is a primetime weekly talk show that airs on Metro Television on Friday nights. It has been airing on television since 2002, in the beginning as Thank God Its Friday (TGIF).

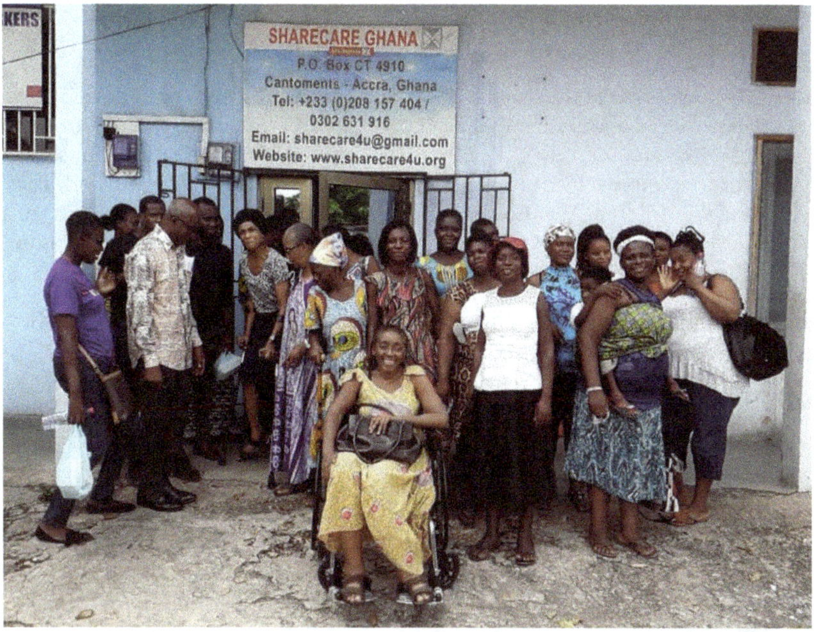
SHARECARE GHANA
P.O. Box CT 4910
Cantonments - Accra, Ghana
Tel: +233 (0)208 157 404 /
0302 631 916
Email: sharecare4u@gmail.com
Website: www.sharecare4u.org

Figure 7.1 Nana Yaa Agyeman with ShareCare Ghana members.

disabilities.[11] SCG received funding from GFD for operational costs and from donor partners such as USAID for advocacy activities. They partnered with national institutions on research, education and advocacy. With the Noguchi Memorial Institute for Medical Research (NMIMR), they collaborated on a study to map the epidemiology of neurological disorders in Ghana. They engaged with the Ministry of Health to review and expand the NHIS medicines list to include medications for autoimmune and neurological conditions. They advocated for environmental adjustments in schools for disabled children using a shared platform with the Ministry of Gender, Children and Social Protection (MOGCSP).

ShareCare Ghana operated from an office space in the Accra suburb of Adabraka, at a location that served as a mini-campus for some of GFD's member organisations (Figure 7.1). They also acquired additional space at

[11] The GFD website presents the membership list as: "Ghana Blind Union; Ghana National Association of the Deaf; Ghana Society of the Physically Disabled; Ghana Association of Persons with Albinism; Mental Health Society of Ghana; Inclusion Ghana – a group of people with intellectual disability; Share Care Ghana – a group of people with autoimmune and neurological disorders; Burns Survivors Association – survivors of various degrees of burns; Ghana Stammering Association – persons with various levels of speech impediment" (visit: https://gfd.org.gh).

a centre in Osu, a neighbouring suburb, where free physiotherapy sessions were provided to children.

CA: "So that's one of the flagship activities that Sharecare has been doing which has relieved a lot of families because when they come there, sometimes the children are in a very critical state, but after a few months, you can see a massive improvement in the lives of the kids. We provide assistive devices for the children. We did a cardboard project, where we used the cards to develop some assistive devices for the parents, so that when they are home, they can take care of their children."

Both Nana Yaa Agyeman and Christopher Agbeba ran SCG while they negotiated debilitating illness.

NYA: At the moment I am in a wheelchair, don't have sight in my left eye and I have just regained use of my hands. I don't have the full strength of both hands. On a typical day, I need help getting out of bed to be transferred to a wheelchair and then I go to the bathroom. Fortunately, I am able to do a lot of things in the bathroom but I still need help with my back because I can't stand in the bathroom. From there I go back to the bedroom and I am helped with everything. I can use my hands now so I can feed myself, thankfully. I am wheeled to the living room and I watch a lot of TV even though I don't have full sight at least I can take in the sound. I can't read now, that's something I find a little bit difficult because I love books but at least with technology I can use my computer. I can zoom it up to a full sight and I can get a lot of stuff from the internet. It is manageable, one will wish for more independence but at least we manage from one day to the next.

CA: Sometimes you are dealing with something really painful, you just want the pain to go away. I have nerve cramps, so sometimes I go to bed as early as 9pm, I'm on my bed, but I sleep at 1am. Because that four hours is a banter, it is a fight. [The pain is] uncomfortable. It's a mixture of the deep, sharp and sometimes heat. And *you* would understand that these kinds of conditions also lead to a lot of mental health conditions.

They managed the daily physical pain and psychological struggles by imagining alternative realities through the 'gift of daydreaming' and music.

NYA: I keep telling people God has given me a gift of daydreaming, so instead of living in the moment, I live outside the moment, if that makes any sense. I am able to imagine myself running, kicking, and doing all sort of things and it doesn't keep me down that I am sitting in a wheelchair.

CA: Sometimes just to go through what I go through, I alter reality. Like, I love music a lot so sometimes I consume it. It is like dope. I just consume it.

The daily disruptions were placed within the context of crippling structural barriers faced by SCG members and people living with chronic diseases more generally. They detailed the problems of biomedical care, from the delays in diagnosing neurological conditions – which they had experienced themselves – to the prohibitive cost of medicines.

NYA: With a lot of these conditions, you need the diagnostics, you may need an MRI [Magnetic Resonance Imaging] or a CT [Computed Tomography] scan, which are expensive. In ShareCare, for example, a lot of the members haven't even received diagnosis because they can't afford it. And the NHIS (*National Health Insurance Scheme*) doesn't cover the diagnosis neither does it cover the drugs. So even if you get the diagnosis, you don't have access to the drugs because the drugs are expensive.

Despite a Persons with Disability Act, passed in 2006, which placed emphasis on environmental inclusion, buildings and public transportation were not disability accessible. Nana Yaa Agyeman recalled a meeting with a company that had imported a fleet of buses for public transport:

> We [*SCG*] went to meet the management [of the company], to find out if the buses were accessible and we found out only two of the new buses were wheelchair accessible. The management was asking us which route we will suggest those two buses ply? And we said, we can't decide which areas will have persons with disability: they are all over the country.

When Ghana NCD Alliance was established in 2017, Christopher Agbeba was invited to speak at national events and eventually progressed to the global stage as an advocate and peer educator for the Global NCD Alliance.

> There was a period where I really struggled with self-esteem trying to really understand what was going on, because here is the case where a lot of my mates are going to school. They are looking forward to the bigger things in life to achieve. I'm looking forward to [. . .] I don't know what. So, it was ShareCare that put me in that position where they said 'you can be very impactful'. Nana Yaa helped me get a job and I started working. Then I realized that I was being very productive in terms of meetings, events and being able to speak publicly. So I was then given the opportunities to do that. Cerebral Palsy Day, I was speaking and I was seated by Zenator Rawlings[12] and for me, that was the beginning of me believing that there was something I could offer. And it got to its peak when I got in touch with the NCD Alliance. And this happened through ShareCare again. In 2018, an opportunity came and I travelled to Switzerland to be trained as an advocate. In 2019, I was taken back again to be trained as a peer trainer. In 2020, before COVID had hit Ghana, I also went to the UAE [United

[12] Member of Parliament in Ghana and daughter of former President Jerry John Rawlings. Nana Yaa Agyeman was the younger sister of Nana Konadu Agyeman-Rawlings, wife of Jerry John Rawlings. This fact was well known publicly but was not raised or discussed in her interview.

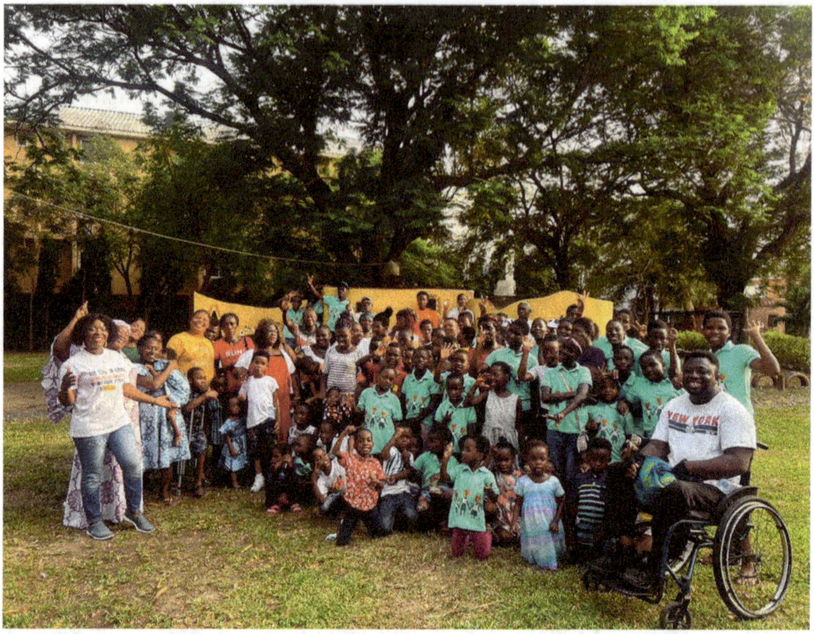

Figure 7.2 Christopher Agbeba with children from SCG and Jamestown Children's Health Club at a Christmas party in December 2023.

> Arab Emirates]. There was a conference, the NCD Alliance forum, where I also spoke. I went with the current minister for Oti region, Mr. Joshua Makubu. It was also a very impactful session.

Through the opportunities provided by SCG and the NCD Alliance, Christopher Agbeba had told his story on the global stage and "travelled across the country, trained people and become an advocate" (see Figure 7.2). He had become conscientised and experienced self-transformation: journeying from feelings of low self-esteem to recognising he could be 'very impactful'. This personal change did not translate to group-level change, however. During the first year of the COVID-19 pandemic – months after his UAE conference panel sharing experience with a local MP – SCG "was kicked out of the centre" (Agbeba) they had used for children's physiotherapy sessions. Despite the government's recognition of higher COVID-19 risks for individuals with underlying chronic conditions, no special allowances were made for patient groups.

Throughout SCG's existence, group level change had come from the ingenuity, social creativity and hard work of the group's leader and members, and from support provided by the group's local and international allies. "One interesting thing about Ghana", Christopher Agbeba observed, "is that it has a lot of policies but you don't see implementation." Nana Yaa Agyeman laid the blame on a dereliction of duty by political leaders:

> I think it is a matter of prioritizing and a matter of interest. I mean our so-called leaders, they travel and see what happens in the so-called developed world, they admire it, and they come back and do nothing about the issues here.

The Scope and Limits of NCD Stories

By the time SCG was established in 2007, there were several patient support groups for NCDs across the country (de-Graft Aikins et al., 2010; see Table 7.1). Some of these groups pre-dated SCG by a decade: the first patient support group, Ghana Diabetes Association, was established in the late 1990s.

Pedrinho Guareschi and Sandra Jovchelovitch (2004), following Paulo Freire, define conscientisation in the context of community health development as a "process through which critical thinking develops" and in terms of "a politics and a psychology of recognition where otherwise socially excluded subjects come into the public arena to state who they are, what they know and what they want". SCG and other patient support groups were conscientised: through their publicly disclosed personal and group stories they "state[d] who they were, what they knew and what they wanted" in relation to their shared "life-disrupting problems" (Katz, 1981). They forged productive alliances with caregivers, healthcare professionals, local and international civil society groups and other allies. They amplified the impact of their personal and shared stories through concrete actions – marches to raise awareness, fundraising, lobbying government sector ministries and policymakers, and collaborating on research (Figure 7.3).

But like SCG, patient support groups have faced multilayered challenges. Firstly, there are physical and mental limits to doing advocacy while living with a chronic illness or being a caregiver. Secondly, funding challenges are constantly negotiated: a number of the pioneering groups that were operating in the early 2000s folded due to lack of funds. Thirdly, cultural barriers persist: people living with conditions that are poorly understood and stigmatised in society, such as breast cancer and dementia, find disclosure difficult, even within safe spaces of support groups. Finally,

Table 7.1 *Selected patient support groups for chronic diseases in Ghana.*

Condition	Advocacy group	Type
Alzheimer's disease and dementia	Alzheimer's Ghana	Expert (doctor) led
Autoimmune and neurological conditions	Share Care Ghana	Peer (patient) led
Cancers	Breast Care International	Peer (doctor) led
	DWIB Leukaemia Trust	Peer (patient) led
	Ghana Parents Association for Childhood Cancer	Peer (caregiver) led Peer (caregiver) led
	Lifeline for Childhood Cancer	Peer (survivor) led
	Reach for Recovery	Expert led
	Run for a Cure	
Cardiovascular and heart disease	Ghana Heart Foundation	Expert led
	Jamestown Health Club*	Expert (psychologist) led
Diabetes	Ghana Diabetes Association	Expert-Peer led
Endometriosis	Endo Charity	Peer (patient) led
Lupus	Oyemam Autoimmune Foundation	Peer (patient) led
Mental illness	Basic Needs Ghana*	Expert led (NGO)
	Mental Health Society of Ghana (MEHSOG)	Expert led (NGO) Expert led (NGO)
	Mindfreedom Ghana	
Parkinsons disease	Parkinson's Disease Support Group	Expert (physiotherapist) led
Rare diseases	Rare Disease Ghana Initiative	Expert led (NGO)
Rheumatoid arthritis	Resolute Initiative	Expert (physician) led
Stroke	Stroke Association Support Network	Expert-peer led

*Some groups and organisations deal with more than one condition. Basic Needs provides support for individuals and families affected by epilepsy in addition to mental illness. Jamestown Health Club was established following a study on cardiovascular disease (CVD) experiences in Ga Mashie (see de-Graft Aikins, 2020), but members also live with diabetes and post-stroke conditions. This list is not exhaustive, as it is based on groups with a sustained public presence and web or social media profiles.

structural barriers restrict access to timely and accurate diagnoses, affordable medicines and medical technologies, and continuity of care.

At a general level, the OVOV project complemented the pre-existing culture of NCD advocacy through storytelling. By telling their personal stories on television or radio, at community events or at national

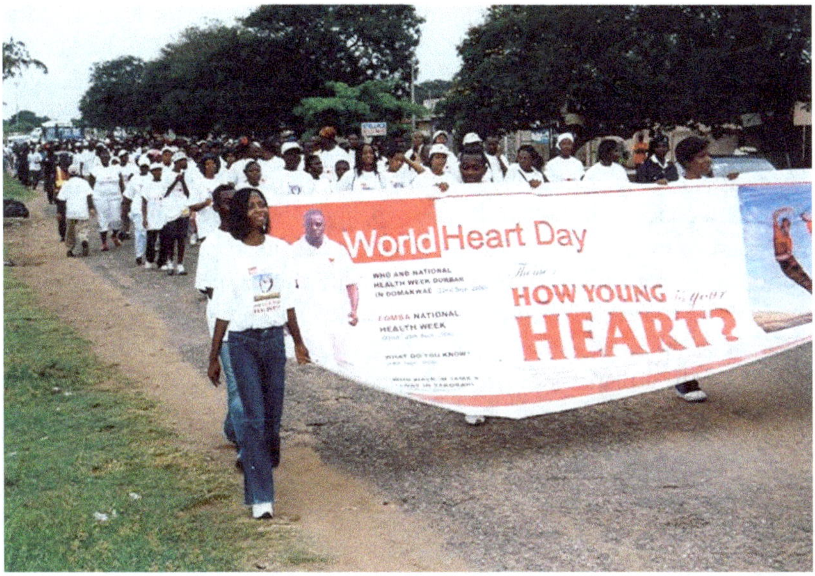

Figure 7.3 Marching for World Hypertension Day.

conferences, NCD advocates increased lay awareness and understanding of specific chronic diseases and of chronic illness experiences more generally. Agbeba's understanding of his own health condition began with seeing Agyeman tell her story on a popular television show. Furthermore, storytelling sharpened their advocacy skills and led to self-transformation.

The Alliance's first goal of using stories to 'take charge' was achieved, albeit with a limited set of workshopped narratives. But NCD confessional technologies – like the HIV versions – were also political technologies: they reproduced unequal forms of power between individuals and agencies that required, or benefited from, the confessions. This undermined the Alliance's second goal of 'driving change'. This point is illustrated by examining the critical considerations of narrative health.

Who was telling the stories? People living in three cities who were fluent English speakers. The strategy of locating workshops in three cities and limiting the language of instruction to English excluded a wide swathe of participants across the country who may have had stories to tell in any of Ghana's forty-plus local languages.

How were they telling the stories? In a pre-determined standard format imposed during the workshops, which failed to factor in cultural norms around illness disclosure. Telling stories of chronic illness can be a double-edged sword in Ghanaian communities. As we saw in Ruth's story (Chapter 2) and with Yankah's (2004) AIDSlore narratives (Chapter 4), despite the cultural imperative to 'sell one's sickness', doing so is fraught with psycho-spiritual dangers. Therapy damagers might be operating at the interpersonal level. Stigma may develop and spread at the community level. After careful reflection of why the story must be told in the first place, one must then choose who to tell the story to, and when, where and how to tell the story. Stigma consciousness was a cross-cutting theme in the featured stories of the four NCD advocates. The reluctance of people to sign up to the OVOV project was associated with these sociocultural factors.

What communities benefited from the shared stories? By disseminating the stories on the Alliance website and social media platforms, in English, it appeared that the beneficiaries of the OVOV project were global (English-speaking) audiences and not local actors. In her story, Ama Quainoo pointed out the limitations of English language based health education in Ghanaian communities:

> During our awareness raising activities on COVID-19 and NCDs and their risk factors, some communities [found] it difficult to understand our messages and vice-versa due to different dialects. Access to information is our fundamental right. We hope plenty of information regarding NCDs in different dialects and languages will be made available.

British sociologists Imogen Tyler and Tom Slater (2018), writing about anti-stigma mental health campaigns, note that global mental health charities and organisations co-opt and sanitise the "sharing of testimonies [which] has long been a central strategy of grassroots mental health activism, particularly in struggles against 'psychiatric authority'". They "mobilise an array of communications technologies, developing a website, harnessing social media platforms (Facebook, Twitter and Instagram), and devising hashtags [. . .] under which people can share their experiences". The audiences for these stories are not those living with or affected by mental illness, but "powerful corporate, charity and government actors" (p.724). Ultimately, their campaign strategies serve corporate interests but "do little to change the way that agencies function or to address broader causes of mental distress and mental illness such as poverty, unemployment and discrimination" (p.724).

Historically, policy responses to the growing burden of NCDs in Ghana have been slow and discontinuous. After the establishment of the Non-communicable Disease Control Programme (NCDCP) in the late 1990s, two attempts have been made to develop a policy. The first, funded by

MOH, was a homegrown five-year multi-stakeholder process led by William Bosu, the NCDCP programme manager at the time, which led to an official launch in 2012 (Bosu, 2012). The second attempt, funded by the World Bank, convened a different set of stakeholders and leaders, including external experts with links to the NCD Alliance, and led to an official relaunch in 2019. Both policies applied a "whole of government, whole of society" (WoG, WoS) approach – a new framework developed in 2011, when the United Nations convened its first high-level meeting on NCDs in New York.

> WoG is an approach 'in which public service agencies work across portfolio boundaries' to develop integrated policies and programmes towards the achievement of shared or complementary, interdependent goals. WoS mov[es] beyond public authorities and engag[es] 'all relevant stakeholders, including individuals, families and communities, intergovernmental organizations, religious institutions, civil society, academia, the media, voluntary associations and [. . .] the private sector and industry' (Ortenzi et al., 2022, p.1).

At the centre of the WoS goals was empowering 'individuals, families and communities' to take charge of their health, partly because low- and middle-income countries (LMIC) health systems were grappling with complex health disease burdens with limited human and financial resources. As previous sections show, individuals, families and communities affected by NCDs in Ghana had been taking charge of their health, through the advocacy of patient support groups, decades before the 2011 UNHLM. But the greatest barrier to personal and social change consistently emerged from the WoG end of the relationship. The implementation of NCD policies has not worked across portfolio boundaries and through integrated policies and programmes: pre-existing policies on mental health, disability and active ageing, for example, remain separate from the NCD policy (Alidu et al., 2016; Bosu, 2012; de-Graft Aikins et al., 2021).

The NCD Alliance storytelling project entered an already problematic space of performative policymaking, which was well known to patient support groups. As Christopher Agbeba observed: "Ghana [. . .] has a lot of policies but you don't see implementation." Nii Sampa, Sister Aku and other Jamestown Health Club members did not believe sharing personal stories would change their life circumstances.

The challenge patient support groups have faced for decades is to tell stories that do not only highlight the 'slow violence' of living with chronic illness under conditions of prolonged policy inaction but also have the conscientising force to change the way policymakers and other powerful political actors address the social and structural causes and consequences of chronic conditions. This is an impossible challenge.

Policy inaction on NCDs is driven by long-standing health governance flaws. Ghana's health system was built in the colonial era when the prevalent conditions were infectious. Although the country's health profile has changed, with populations facing complex disease burdens, healthcare models and health policies are ideologically oriented towards privileging time-limited treatment over prevention and long-term illness management. This ideological position affects all areas of the healthcare system, from building an appropriate workforce, through procurement of medicines and technologies, to developing inclusive health insurance. This problem is further compounded by the over-reliance of government actors on 'donor partners', who by financing health and other areas of social life, also set the terms for naming, understanding and addressing local health problems. Because of these powerful ideological, financial and political factors, changing the health policy environment through the arts requires more radical methods.

Lucy Costa and colleagues (2012) describe a project they developed called 'Hands Off Our Stories', which used a blend of facts, humour and wearable paraphernalia to teach members of their Canadian mental health collective to withhold their stories from exploitative global health actors, to consider telling stories "in a way that is politically accountable and focused on social justice change" (p.99), and to use their limited energies and resources to organise for equitable and culturally appropriate mental health services. The strategy employed in this project involved people working around political authority using socially creative methods. This strategy is well honed in Ghanaian communities, is often deployed to counter structural violence, and can inform new approaches to NCD advocacy that amplify the strengths of storytelling and buffer its weaknesses with alternative creative responses.

CHAPTER 8

Colonial Virus

Ghanaian comedian and actor Clemento Suarez (real name Clement Ashitey) posted a comedy sketch that went viral on Ghanaian social media in March 2020, just days after a three-week COVID-19 lockdown was imposed on Accra, Kumasi and selected communities on the outskirts of both cities. In the video – a parody of the media vox pop – Suarez played a schoolboy called Timothy, who was walking along the road in the standard-issue brown and beige school uniform for public schools when he was stopped by a female journalist.

"Aha, Timothy, tell me the corona ABCD", the journalist said in Twi, thrusting a microphone in Timothy's face.

"Hehe, Colonial ABCD", Timothy smirked before launching into his recital.

As schoolboy Timothy worked his way through the "Colonial ABCDs", he told a funny but thoughtful and complex story of the early impact of the COVID-19 pandemic in Ghana (similar to the visual story told in Chaotic COVID-19, Figure 8.1). Each alphabet covered a topical COVID-19 theme, ingeniously rendered in a blend of Twi, Twinglish and English (see full sketch in Appendix 3d). He covered prevention themes (H) and the responses of religious leaders to the pandemic (O). In a nod to global affairs (E), he inserted a line on King (then Prince) Charles' bout of COVID-19 in the early months of the pandemic. Suarez also evoked collective memories of past national hardships, such as the curfews of the 1970s military coup years presided over by former president Jerry John Rawlings (J) and the 1983 famine (T). He ended with a sarcastic shout-out to the Zongo Minister (Z) – a new and controversial ministerial portfolio established by the NPP government that aimed, but had failed, to address poverty in urban migrant communities.

The creative impact of the sketch was all down to Suarez's comedic skill. But the content of his sketch was as much a function of this skill as it was the function of the creativity of social responses to COVID-19.

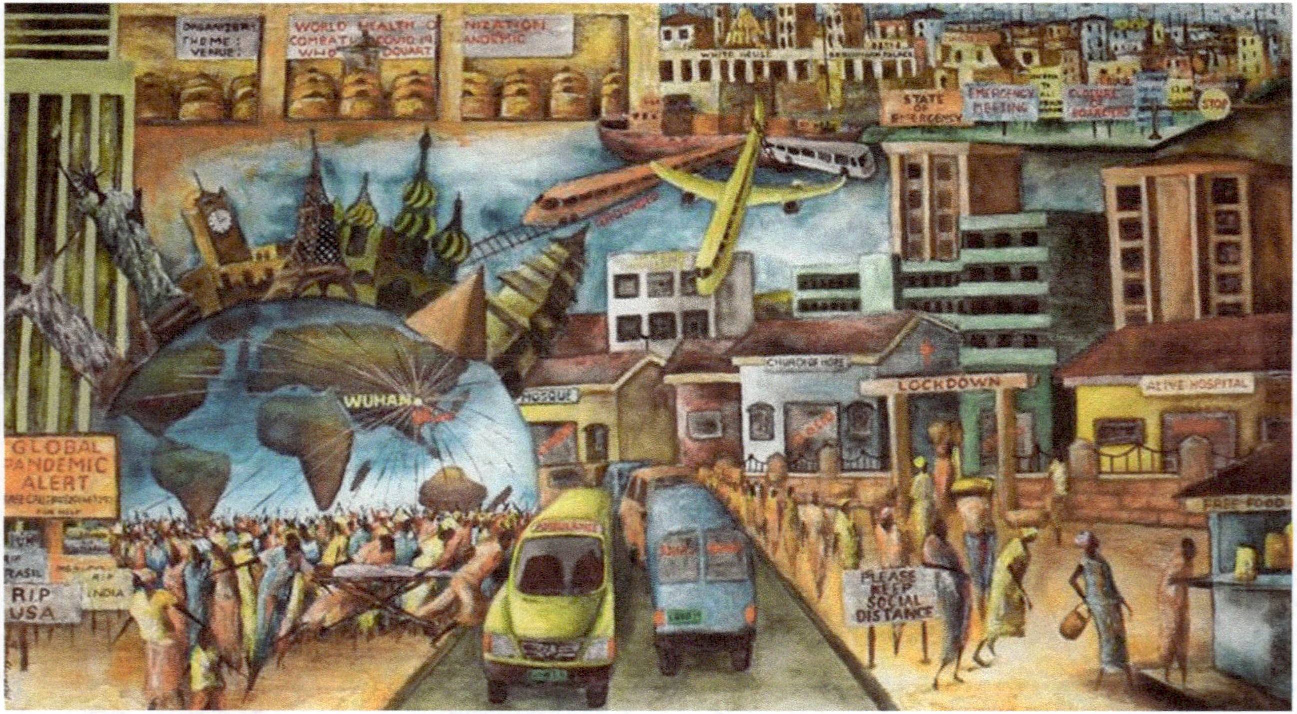

Figure 8.1 Chaotic COVID-19, painting by Agyei Agyemang, 2021. Author's collection.

The first two cases of COVID-19 arrived in Ghana's capital, Accra, on 12 March 2020 via international air passengers from endemic Asian and European countries. Early hospital admissions and deaths were linked to underlying chronic conditions. Initially perceived as a far-flung problem of China and Europe, COVID-19 became a domestic problem; but even then, it was perceived as a problem for a privileged urban class, who lived with a higher risk of chronic diseases and had the means to travel. The term *esikafo yareɛ* (disease of the wealthy)[1] became a popular lay theory in poor urban and rural communities.

As local infections spread, a collaborative response to prevention emerged: seamstresses and tailors produced masks with local textiles, local pharmaceutical companies produced hand sanitisers, churches offered spaces for quarantining, and scientists innovated on testing models. At the same time, public understandings and practices developed in ways that mimicked responses to previous public health threats. Even before the government imposed the partial lockdown, traditional and social media had given Ghanaians a taste of what ordinary people were thinking about the pandemic. There were countless vox pops and WhatsApp videos of market women, school children, tro-tro drivers and people going about their daily lives expressing their colourful views and inventive concepts on the new English scientific terms that the Ghana Health Service (GHS) and associated experts used to explain the pandemic: 'coronavirus', 'social distancing', 'respiratory hygiene' and 'superspreader'. Terms blending Pidgin English, local languages, and a blend of English and local languages (e.g., Twinglish, Fantenglish) like 'colona vilus' and 'nose ma' emerged. Interventions were proposed, such as greeting with elbows, ankles and other body parts (Figure 8.2) and using local homebrews, such as *akpeteshie*, as hand sanitisers and stress relievers (Figure 8.3). When Ghana's president, Nana Addo Dankwa Akufo-Addo, began giving regular national addresses on the government's COVID-19 strategy, his standard greeting of 'Fellow Ghanaians' joined the multi-lingual lexicon of COVID-19 satire. These "localized terminologies" (Barz and Cohen, 2011) of COVID-19 were laced with humour – a strategy usually deployed by Ghanaians as a coping strategy when confronted with the new, unsettling or grotesque.[2]

[1] This was also a theme in South Africa, see Sitto and Lubinga (2020).

[2] This strategy, it should be noted, is neither unique to Ghanaians nor a new phenomenon. Humour was employed to cope with Cholera in nineteenth-century Britain (Park and Park, 2010) and with the Spanish flu in the United States (Foss, 2020). As the COVID-19 pandemic progressed, humour became a strategy in many countries, as seen through viral social media posts. In the United Kingdom and United States, COVID-19 comedy stars like Munya Chawawa and Sarah Cooper were born (see Kale, 2021 and Li, 2020).

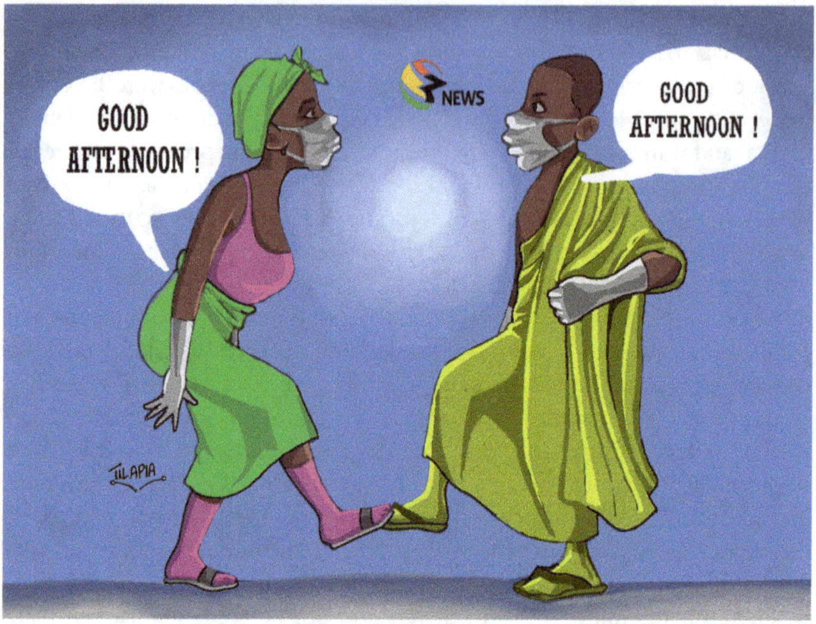
GOOD AFTERNOON !
GOOD AFTERNOON !
NEWS
TILAPIA

Figure 8.2 Coronavirus Greetings, cartoon by Tilapia da Cartoonist, March 2020.

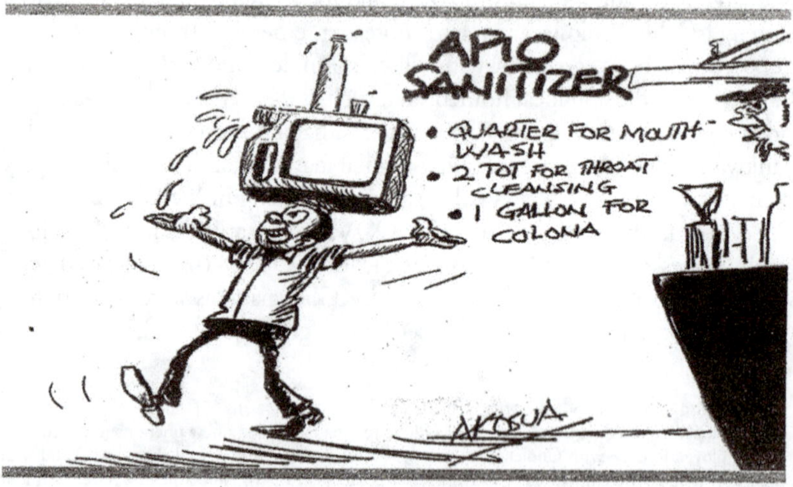
APIO SANITIZER
• QUARTER FOR MOUTH WASH
• 2 TOT FOR THROAT CLEANSING
• 1 GALLON FOR COLONA
AKOSUA

Figure 8.3 Apio Sanitiser, cartoon by Akosua, March 2020.

The humour did not mask a growing fear of the new pandemic, however: social practices told a different story. As community spread established, COVID-19 stigma and stigma consciousness emerged in ways that mimicked HIV/AIDS experiences: fear of infection, of testing and of disclosing test results, for instance. Stigma consciousness, at a collective level, also manifested in conspiracy theories – circulated on social media and in church sermons – about the development of anti-African COVID-19 vaccines in Western laboratories.

Herbalists and religious leaders promoted cures for COVID-19, just as they had offered cures for the Spanish flu, yellow fever and AIDS decades prior (de-Graft Aikins, 2020, Scott, 1965). People experimented with these 'cures', but also adapted existing home remedies for colds, fevers and malaria. They also kept their ears to the ground for new remedies across pluralistic healthcare systems. When a group of local scientists circulated a new, untested theory on WhatsApp about the preventive benefits of hydrogen peroxide – based on their rapid response letter to the *British Medical Journal*[3] – local pharmacies in Accra ran out of stock, and the Community Practice Pharmacy Association issued a communiqué on social media.

A new genre of 'COVID-19 arts' emerged as creative arts communities captured and translated the science, culture and politics of the pandemic for Ghanaian communities at home and abroad. In the sections that follow, I will outline the methods I used to define and track COVID-19 arts, detail their communicative functions, and reflect on insights these new art forms present for pandemic health communication.

'COVID Arts' – Defining and Tracking a New Genre

During the first year of the pandemic, I was interested in the intersections between COVID-19 and chronic conditions and evolving social responses to these in Ghanaian communities (de-Graft Aikins, 2020). The spontaneous artistic responses afforded the opportunity to examine in real-time, how grassroots arts and bottom-up social responses to health crises influenced pandemic health communication. Working with a local team, we tracked these COVID-19 arts in the first year and beyond, as the pandemic evolved through significant phases – vaccine development, vaccine deployment, the evolution of major new variants such as Delta and Omicron – and engendered new social responses. We gathered data from traditional media (newspapers), social media (Twitter now X, Instagram,

[3] See Ayettey et al. (2020).

Facebook, WhatsApp) and public spaces in Accra and Kumasi. We tracked these art forms and emerging genres in real-time – expanding the range of sources to include healthcare spaces such as hospitals, biomedical and herbal clinics, pharmacies and chemical shops.

I defined 'COVID art' as any type of single or multi-form artistic expression that incorporated themes on the COVID-19 pandemic. COVID-19 themes included expert and lay knowledge and representations. I defined experts as those working in health, health policy and allied professions who officially produced and disseminated official COVID-19 information in public forums or for their specialist communities – these included basic scientists (e.g., virologists, biochemists), epidemiologists, medical doctors, pharmacists, public health researchers, economists, psychologists and other social scientists, as well as government ministers officially tasked to communicate to the public on COVID-19. I included indigenous healing systems under the expert category – and specifically herbalists, shrine priests and Christian pastors. In the expert domain, I focused on public health (e.g., 'social distancing', 'test and trace'), social science and policy terms (e.g., 'COVID relief fund'). I defined lay people as ordinary citizens in Ghana living and working outside these expert domains.[4] In the lay domain, I was interested in 'creative practices of the imagination'. Ghanaians engaged with global responses to the pandemic, from its early days (as seen through Suarez's reference to COVID-19 threats in the British Royal Family). Responses from scientific experts, political leaders and ordinary citizens around the world permeated local representations of COVID-19 via traditional and social media, as well as diaspora family and social networks. These global perspectives were included in my definition and examination of local responses.

Based on this definition, seven COVID art forms were identified: cartoons, comedy, fashion (masks), funerary arts, murals, songs and textiles. The database of COVID arts, from January 2020 to the time of writing (October 2023), consists of comedy sketches, cartoons by three political cartoonists (Tilapia da Cartoonist, Akosua and Makaveli), songs in six genres (Dirge, Highlife, Hiplife, Reggae, Gospel, Folk Song), photographs of murals (painted in suburbs in Accra), textile designs by Ghana Textiles Printing (GTP), assorted masks produced locally from African print fabrics by local seamstresses based in Accra and Kumasi, images produced by one group of dancing pallbearers called Nana Otafrija Pallbearing and Waiting Services, a painting of the COVID-19 story in

[4] Although it is important to note that individuals within the expert domain can be categorised as lay in areas of COVID-19 science and policy for which they have no technical expertise.

Ghana (acquired from the Artists Alliance Gallery in Accra) (Figure 8.1), and COVID-19 – themed herbal medicine packaging and advertising.

The analysis of COVID arts was underpinned by two questions: What art and health functional domains did these art forms occupy? What were the social psychological mechanisms through which they operated? The majority of COVID art forms channelled and/or amplified 'creative practices of the imagination' regarding COVID-19, highlighting a mutually constitutive relationship between lay responses to the pandemic and what artists produced. COVID arts functioned in three arts and health domains: health education and knowledge production (creating awareness, evoking memory, conscientising), disease prevention, and (indirectly) to COVID-19 policy development. Almost every art form functioned in more than one domain. These intersecting functions converged on the science, culture and politics of COVID-19.

"Stay Home or Dance with Us": Communicating the Science of COVID-19

All the art forms, except textile designs, focused on handwashing, social distancing, mask-wearing and the various COVID-19 precautions advocated by the GHS.

The prevention themes were covered in songs produced in all the genres aimed at diverse communities across Ghana.[5] Singers applied the 'edutainment' approach. The majority of COVID-19 songs were produced independently by artists. There was one exception. Kofi Kinaata, an award-winning Highlife artist, produced a Highlife song titled 'Coronavirus' that was funded by USAID in collaboration with the University of Rhode Island, government sector ministries and national fishing advocacy organisations.[6] The song targeted Ahanta, Ewe, Fante and Ga fishing communities along Ghana's southern coast. It had a catchy melody and funny lyrics, delivered in Pidgin English, Ahanta, Ewe, Fante and Ga.

Verse 1 (Fante)

Coronavirus, COVID-19	Corona Virus, COVID-19
Mennfa ndi agorɔ koraa ooh	This virus is dangerous,
Wɔ yɛ huu	don't joke with it.
Wo ayɛ merɛ, Fever na ɛbɔbɔ wo, w'abrɛ	The symptoms are fever and coughing, tiredness,
Wo ho na ɛdodɔ dodɔ wo	high temperature,
Ɛbɛ hwɛ ɛnti scent, ɛnti taste	loss of smell and taste;

[5] See examples in Appendix 3. [6] See Appendix 3a for full details.

Wo minemu ye wo yaa ooh, ɛntu mi ndzidzi	sore throat, loss of appetite.
Ɛbɛ rani na ɛnya cold Ɛntumi ngye ahome oh, e feeli dizzy Ɔyɛ hu papaa Yaliba ye wasiɛ bɛɛ bia	You'll experience running stomach and cold, shortness of breath and feeling dizzy. It's very scary! This pandemic has destroyed a lot in the world.
Asia wa kukumu nipa Europe wa gugu ndwuma Na Africa nso di agoro a, asem bɛ ba, hwɛ	In Asia it has killed multitudes Even in Europe it has collapsed corporations. So in Africa if we handle it with levity, it'll overwhelm us.
Refrain Soldier suro corona Lawyer ɔsuro corona Mallam suro corona Wa la wo pastor yi ɔsuro corona	 The soldier is terrified of corona The Lawyer is terrified of corona The Mallam is terrified of corona Even your own pastor is terrified of corona.
Chorus Nia ye hu, nia y'ati, nti obia suro corona Nia ye hu ooh, nia y'ati yen nyinaa yɛ suro corona Nti wo nso suro corona	**Chorus** Because of what we've witnessed and heard, we are terrified of corona. Because of what we've witnessed and heard, we are all terrified of corona. So you should also be terrified of Corona
Verse 2 Hyɛ wo nose mask sɛ ɛrekɔ kurom a Men ma wo werɛ nfi wo two meters, Social distance wo ɛpo no na no Hohoro wo nsa fa samina yɛ Hand sanitizer no fa bi fa yɛɛ Men taa mpuwepuwe Eni hwee yɛ a, n'atena fie Seisei deɛ yen kyimakyima, by heart Yɛn kyima mpo na yɛ hyia hyia, aha Yɛn hyia mpo na yɛ kyia kyia Nti gyae kasa tintin na twa ne tietia ko fie	 Wear your nose mask when you're going out Don't forget the two meter social distancing at the seashore. Wash your hands with soap, And don't forget to use hand sanitizers If you don't have anything relevant to do out, stay home. Irrelevant outing is now a thing of the past So don't go out to exchange pleasantries So keep the long conversations short and go home

The accompanying video was professionally produced and directed by Ghanaian music video director Abass. It was set on a coastal location, with shots of the beach and ocean, of Kinaata dancing to the verses and standing behind a lectern singing the prevention messages into large microphones with local media logos, while wearing a white t-shirt branded with a USAID logo. Around him, members of the fishing communities at work and at leisure applied the COVID-19 prevention strategies. Some wore masks while cleaning and smoking fish and mending fishing nets. Some washed their hands after fish work – with prominently displayed Lifebuoy soap bars (produced by Unilever Ghana). Women danced playfully at physical distance, in moves resembling the Fante traditional *apatampa* dance.

The song and video targeted fishing communities specifically – for instance, warnings against maritime crime were incorporated into the lyrics – and the production appeared to be based on long-standing research between the funding and collaborating partners. But Kinaata's unique artistic blend of catchy melodies and choruses, Fante humour, teachable dance moves and colourful visuals set his song apart from others . This multi-form art spoke beyond the target local communities.[7]

In March 2020, the Ghana Graffiti Collective (GCC) painted a mural on COVID-19 prevention in a suburb of Accra (Figure 8.4). Their work was supported by the Accra Metropolitan Assembly (AMA), the International Organization for Migration (IOM) and the Delegation of the European Union (EU) in Ghana. The mural performed an educational function by featuring the core COVID-19 prevention messages. But it also served aesthetic functions. Painted as a panoramic visual image and story in vivid colours of yellow, blue, burgundy and green, the mural improved the aesthetics of the public environment. It covered the typical patchwork of posters, leaflets and warning signs that cover public walls in major cities. Similar murals were painted in communities across the country with support from the EU, UNICEF and other donor partners.

Ghana was the first African country to receive the first consignment of AstraZeneca vaccines through the COVID-19 Vaccines Global Access (COVAX) Facility in March 2021.[8] Research had reported vaccination

[7] Between 2020 and 2023, I gave guest lectures on 'arts and health communication in African contexts' at the LSE (Health Communication MSc course at the Department of Psychological and Behavioural Science) and Oxford (Translational Science and Global Health MSc Programme run by the Department for Continuing Education), for which I played the Kinaata video as a case study. Students came from the United Kingdom and several other countries, including Australia, Brazil, Canada, India, Nigeria, South Africa and the United States. The video received the same comments across three class cohorts: 'impressive videography', 'rich colours', 'attractive locations (the beach)', 'melody engaging'; 'You feel your legs moving', said Professor Martin Bauer, convenor of the LSE class, in March 2023. However, for students from countries inundated by public health campaigns funded by donor partners – India and Brazil in particular – the initial positive response gave way to criticism about how external funding sources corrupted the authenticity of public health messaging. For some, the prominence given to Lifebuoy soap introduced an ulterior motive.

[8] COVAX is the vaccines pillar of the Access to COVID-19 Tools (ACT) Accelerator. It is described on the GAVI website as a global partnership between GAVI, the Coalition for Epidemic Preparedness Innovations (CEPI), the World Health Organization (WHO) and UNICEF that aims to "accelerate the development and manufacture of COVID-19 vaccines, and to guarantee fair and equitable access for every country in the world".

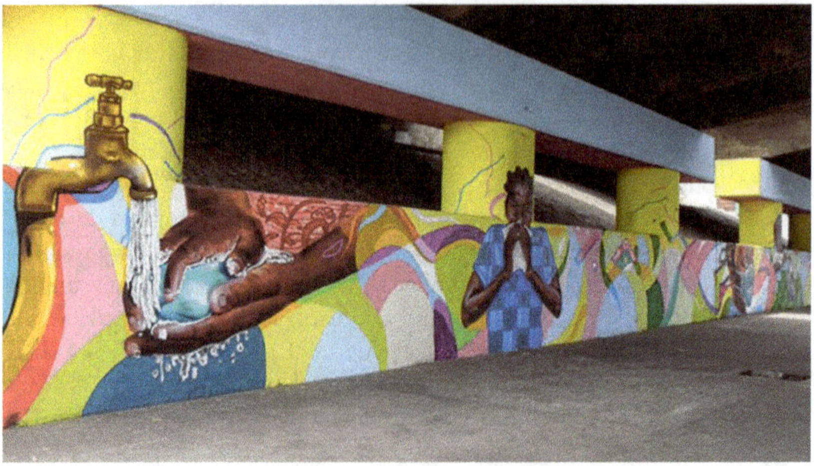

Figure 8.4 COVID-19 mural, painted by Ghana Graffiti Collective, Accra, March 2020 (photograph by Mo Awudu, reproduced with permission).

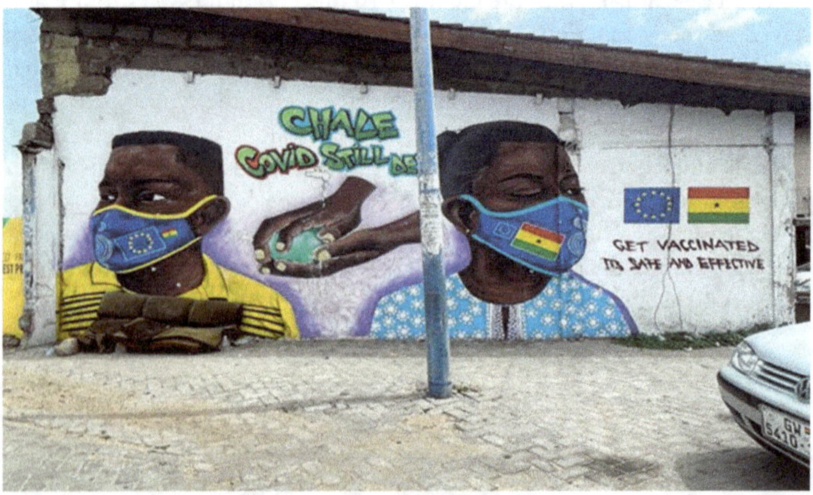

Figure 8.5 "Chale Covid Still De" COVID-19 mural painted by Hamid Nii Nortey April, 2021 (photograph from the author's COVID art database).

hesitancy and resistance in poor urban and rural communities. An intensive drive was initiated to encourage vaccination uptake. In Ga Mashie, an EU-funded COVID-19 mural painted by local artist and muralist Hamid Nii Nortey, in April 2021, focused on messages of mask-wearing, handwashing and vaccination (Figure 8.5).

A creative cottage industry on fashionable masks emerged months before face masks became mandatory in June 2020. Masks produced from waxprint textiles and mask fashion (matching clothing with masks of identical textile designs) were marketed on social media and reached thousands of potential and actual buyers beyond immediate physical social networks (Figure 8.6).

By making masks fashionable and fun, the local mask-making industry facilitated the social adaptation of an uncomfortable but necessary new habit in Ghana, long before other countries like the United Kingdom and United States, which had a higher COVID-19 burden but grappled with the politics and logistics of face coverings (Greenhalgh and de-Graft Aikins, 2023). Masks added a new dimension to Ghanaian fashion

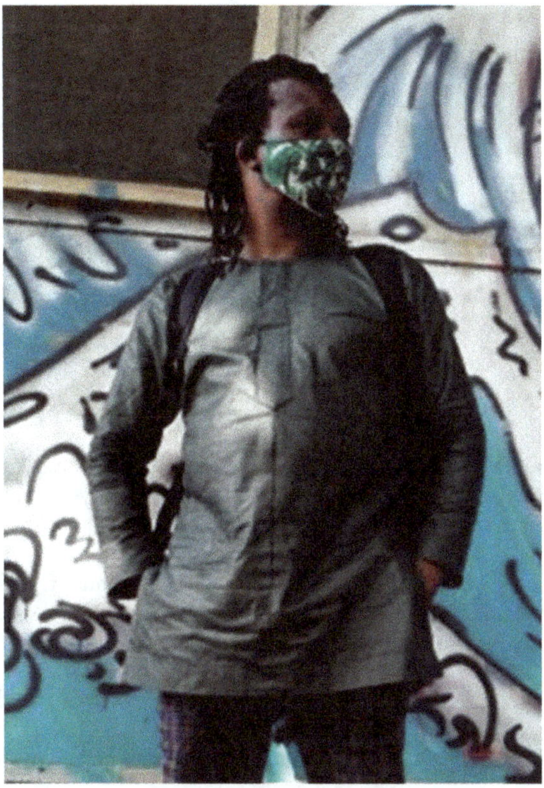

Figure 8.6 Artist and academic Bernard Akoi-Jackson in a face mask made by Jenesus Clothing from batik cotton cloth, Kumasi, Ghana.

aesthetics and also created financial opportunities in a time of economic uncertainty for seamstresses and tailors, as well as more established fashion designers (Osseo-Asare, 2022). These grassroots responses also informed policy decisions on funding local mass production of masks alongside hand sanitisers. In April 2020, the government secured a USD$1 billion loan from the International Monetary Fund (IMF) (IMF, 2020). It was reported – via the president's address to the nation – that this loan would support small businesses and infrastructure development, including building new hospitals in underserved districts. Commitments to small businesses included allocation of funds for local mask production.

Funerary arts in Ghana incorporate various art forms – clay and wood sculpture, textiles, dirges, coffin design and dance – in representing dying, death and the afterlife, and in concrete practices of mourning and commemorating the dead (de Witte, 2011; Parker, 2000; Tschumi and Foster, 2013). The Abibiman group, who specialise in folk songs, composed a COVID-19 prevention song in the mournful tone of a funeral dirge and, like Kinaata, warned that the disease was no respecter of persons. The song was sung in Twi but incorporated Ewe and Ga in the introductory verse.

Corona virus akoadiɛ wuo yi
ɛnya wo aa ɛbe kumwo
ɛde wo bɛkɔ asaman akyere do oooo

Yeee COVID-19 kɔdea wuo yi
Abasen yɛn koomu yi
Yadea yi ɛnya wo aa ɛbɛ ha wo
Yadea yi ɛnya wo aa ebeku wo

Yeee yaanom yadea yi ayɛ hu oo
Yee ɛnsuro obiara ɛnfɛre obiara
Akunini ne abenfo
Ahenfo ne abrempong
Asɔfo ne akɔmfuo
Mallam mpo ka ho bi oo
Asikafo ne ahiafo
Yetu wofo aa wɔntie
COVID-19 na wo kɔfa
Na ede wo bɛ kɔ asaman kyere
do ooo

Coronavirus, that deadly disease
When it gets you, it will kill you
It will take you to the land of the dead

This deadly COVID-19
That has befallen us
When this disease gets you, it will
disturb you

When this disease gets you, it will
kill you
The disease has become scary
It does not fear anyone, nor is it shy
of anyone
Mighty and learned
Kings and Divisional Chiefs
Pastors and Traditional Priests
Even Mallams
The rich and the poor
When we advise you, you don't listen
You will contract COVID-19
And it will take you to the land of the dead

In contrast, Nana Otafrija Pallbearing and Waiting Services (hereafter Nana Otafirija) applied dark humour in their approach to COVID-19 education. Nana Otafrija became a global viral hit in the early months of the pandemic. Their pre-pandemic choreographed dances had already been viewed over a million times across various social media platforms and inspired copycat choreographies and memes on the internet.[9] The pandemic imbued their art with a new meaning, as the imagery they produced joined the global COVID arts landscape (Sullivan, 2020). They coined a darkly humorous message to promote adherence to lock-down measures that struck a chord beyond Ghana and inspired COVID-19 billboard messaging in Brazil: 'stay home or dance with us'.[10]

"What's Up, Fellow Deadly Diseases": Communicating the Culture of COVID-19

In January 2021, actor-comedian Jeffrey Nortey posted a sketch on social media that went viral. In the sketch, coronavirus arrived late to a meeting. "What's up, fellow deadly diseases", coronavirus said, as malaria, cholera and AIDS jumped up from their seats and rushed for their face masks.[11]

Nortey's sketch illustrated one way in which Ghanaians were making sense of the pandemic during its second wave, when infections, hospitalisations and deaths were rising rapidly.[12] While COVID-19 was new and unique then (as it continues to be now), devastating public health threats are long-standing and omnipresent in Ghana. The sketch captured national sentiment about COVID-19 as a familiar alien threat and reflected the emotional tone of social discourse, which had shifted from the light and

[9] See the group head, Benjamin Aidoo's, pinned tweet on the COVID-19 pandemic – @nanaotafrija. In the LSE and Oxford classes, students from South Africa, Brazil and India had seen pre-pandemic and pandemic videos of Nana Otafirija. In Brazil, their image was used in merchandise, such as mugs (LSE class discussion, March 2023).

[10] This message travelled across borders. A Brazilian municipal authority erected billboards with the image of the group and their message. An American journalist observed: "Ghanaian pallbearers dancing with a casket in a highly choreographed routine, lifting it up and lowering it, pretending to drop it and laying down dead in an homage to James Brown, makes all the horrors of the world easier to handle. It's not a joyful laugh, but a grim one" (Jackson, 2020). In April 2022, the group sold one of their iconic dance memes as a non-fungible token (NFT) for a reported $1,047,806 and donated 25 per cent of the proceeds to victims of Russia's war on Ukraine (PR Newswire, 2022).

[11] Visit @jeffreynortey's Instagram page: www.instagram.com/p/CHNTXNtnwo-/?igshid=MDJmNzVkMjY=.

[12] On 2 December 2020, the official number of COVID-19 cases was 51,667. The total number of deaths was 323. There was a spike in hospitalisations and deaths between December and January 2021. This was linked to superspreader events and foreign travel to Ghana; the majority of deaths occurred among older wealthy individuals with histories of chronic conditions such as diabetes and hypertension. Ghana was in tenth place on the top ten list of African countries with the highest number of cases, having occupied fifth place months prior (de-Graft Aikins, 2020).

distanced humour of the early months to macabre humour based on lived experience of infections, stigma, caregiving, job losses and bereavements.

Ghanaian artist El Anatsui observes that “cloth is to the African what monuments are to Westerners” (Walker, 2022, p.50). In Ghana, there is a long-standing tradition of using textiles to memorialise significant family, community and national events. A specific cloth design can be chosen to mourn the death of a family member, or a new cloth design can be commissioned to commemorate a milestone in institutional or national life. When Ghana marked fifty years of independence from British colonial rule in 2007, a new textile design was commissioned to commemorate the national milestone.

In July 2020, Ghana Textiles Printing (GTP) – a Dutch-owned company – built on the tradition of memorialising with textiles by launching new COVID-19 textile designs. The designs featured recognisable symbols of the pandemic: planes for airport closures, padlocks for lockdown, the medical illustration of the coronavirus and, in what appeared to be political homage, the distinctive round eyeglasses worn by Ghana’s president. The new designs captured two iconic events associated with the pandemic. The first, titled ‘Lockdown’ captured the partial lockdown of 2020. This design included padlocks or aeroplanes as a repeated motif. The second, titled ‘Fellow Ghanaians’ captured the president’s addresses to the nation. This incorporated the president’s eye glasses as a repeated motif. For each design, there were two sub-types. The first re-imagined an old classic waxprint design, titled *Odehyie nsu* (A royal does not cry, in Twi) (Figure 8.7). The second was a completely new design (Figure 8.8).

Within weeks of their launch, the new textile designs had captured the attention of global media. In a radio interview with British Broadcasting Corporation (BBC) Focus on Africa, the marketing director of GTP, Stephen Badu, observed:

> We are a business that tells stories and we tell our stories through our designs. [COVID-19] is going to leave a mark in the history of the world, and it’s important that generations that come after us get to know that once upon a time, such a phenomenon occurred.[13]

The annual televised *Ghana’s Most Beautiful* pageant, aired by TV3 Ghana, featured beauty queens wearing designer clothes made with COVID-19 textiles. Political strategists incorporated the textiles into campaign paraphernalia for the December 2020 presidential and parliamentary elections.

[13] Ghanaian COVID-19-inspired fashion print designs launched – BBC News.

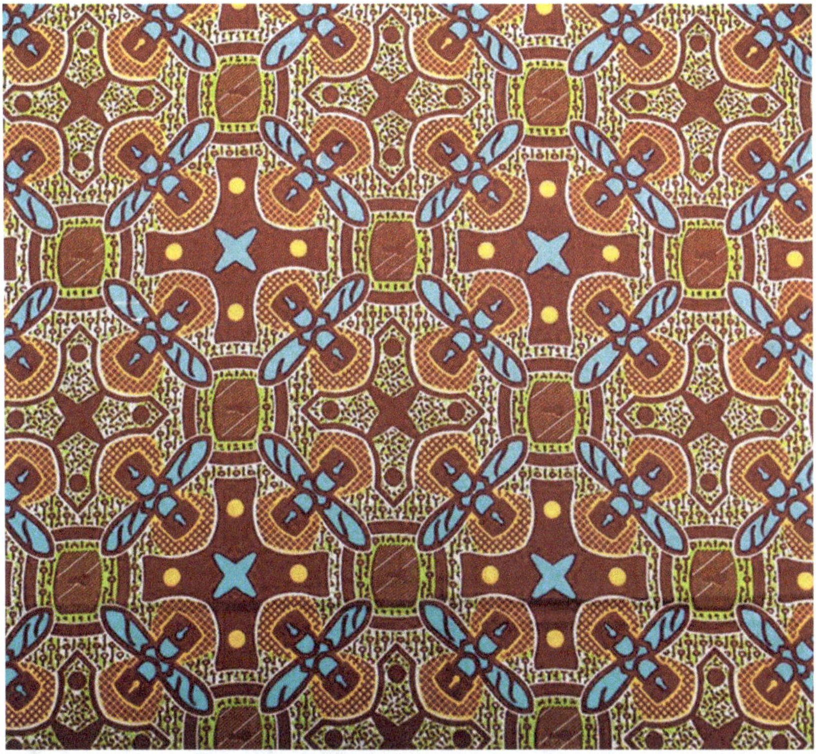

Figure 8.7 'Lockdown', featuring the aeroplane motif, GTP COVID-19 textile design.

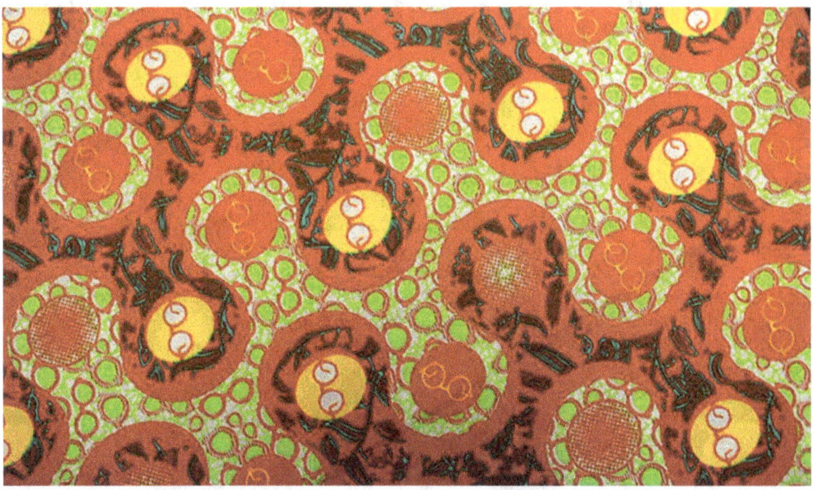

Figure 8.8 'Fellow Ghanaians', featuring the eye glasses motif, GTP COVID-19 textile design.

The designs have now joined the 'Friday Wear' work culture, which encourages workers to support Made in Ghana products by wearing clothing made from locally produced textiles.

"White Man Always Tryna Find Ways": Communicating the Politics of COVID-19

The cartoons produced by Tilapia da Cartoonist, Akosua and Makaveli captured social and political debates on the pandemic. They translated the fears of lay people and social scientists about the economic feasibility of lockdown and social protection for marginalised communities. Tilapia da Cartoonist criticised the short-lived initiative to distribute food to poor and vulnerable communities during lockdown (Figure 8.9), while Makaveli observed the difficulties of eating a balanced diet under financial constraints (Figure 8.10). The cartoonists disputed COVID-19 statistics generated by GHS, even before local research institutions presented evidence that challenged official figures.[14] They predicted the potential misdirection of COVID-19 funds – including the aforementioned IMF loan – by politicians and technocrats. They anticipated economic hardships to come and made comparisons between the 'COVID-19 economy' and the economic impact of the energy crisis Ghana experienced between 2012 and 2016, which Ghanaians creatively christened '*dumsor*' (off and on, in Twi) (Figure 8.11). These artists conscientised their audiences, nudging them towards a critical understanding of the social and political dynamics of COVID-19.[15]

Other artists challenged the global politics of the pandemic response. The hiplife artist Tulenkey performed a song titled "Corona" in English, Pidgin English and Twi. The song covered themes of prevention but also placed the pandemic within the context of preceding pandemics and public health threats (swine flu, HIV and Ebola) and re-presented

[14] Ghana's COVID-19 figures were estimated to be significantly higher than the official statistics during the first year. On 28 October 2020, scientists at the University of Ghana's West African Centre for Cell Biology of Infectious Pathogens (WACCBIP) convened a "Status of COVID-19 in Ghana" webinar. They presented (pre-peer-reviewed) findings of a study with 1,305 individuals that applied a pre-validated antibody rapid diagnostic test (RDT) to determine exposure to the coronavirus. Extrapolations from the WACCBIP study suggested that at least 1.2 million people in Accra (20 per cent of the six million population) had "been infected in the past" (www.wacbip.org/1-million-people-already-exposed-to-COVID-19-in-Accra-scientists-estimate). At the time, the GHS website reported just over 50,000 cases nationally.

[15] Joseph Oduro-Frimpong (2014, p.135), observes that Ghanaian political cartoonists such as Tilapia da Cartoonist, Akosua and Makavelli incorporate "allusions, satire and innuendos in depictions of certain (political) personalities and situations". These depictions carry political weight. Akosua has been sued, unsuccessfully, in the past by a politician who had taken a satirical feature on him quite literally and failed to see the humour. In suing, the politician revealed the inherent subversive and moral power of the political cartoon.

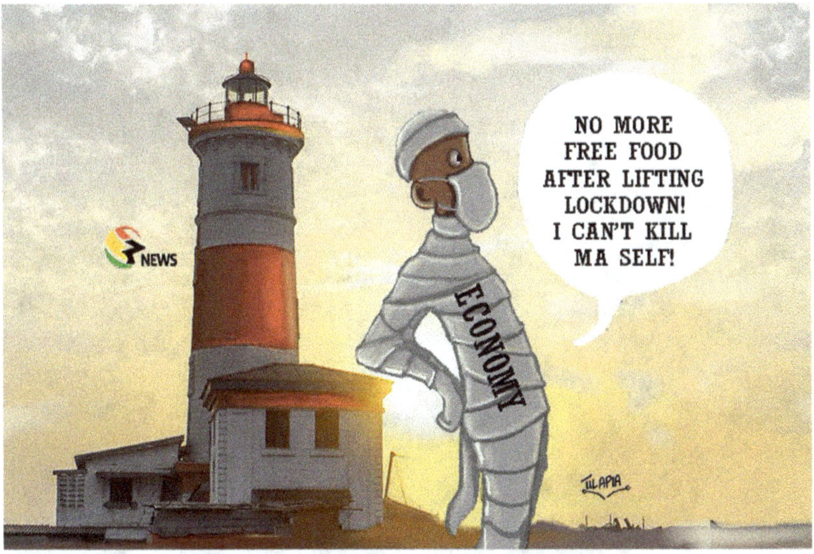
NEWS
NO MORE
FREE FOOD
AFTER LIFTING
LOCKDOWN!
I CAN'T KILL
MA SELF!
ECONOMY
TILAPIA

Figure 8.9 "No more free food after lockdown" cartoon by Tilapia da Cartoonist, April 2020.

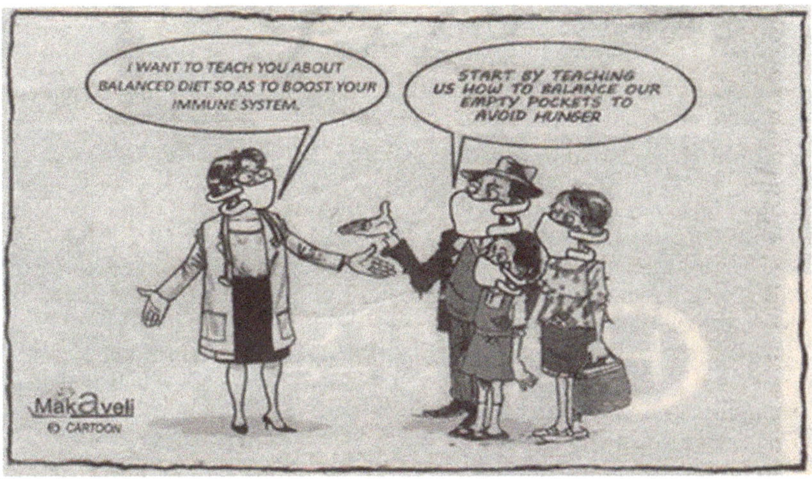
I WANT TO TEACH YOU ABOUT BALANCED DIET SO AS TO BOOST YOUR IMMUNE SYSTEM.
START BY TEACHING US HOW TO BALANCE OUR EMPTY POCKETS TO AVOID HUNGER
Makaveli
© CARTOON

Figure 8.10 'Balanced diet versus balanced pockets' cartoon by Makaveli, 20 April 2020.

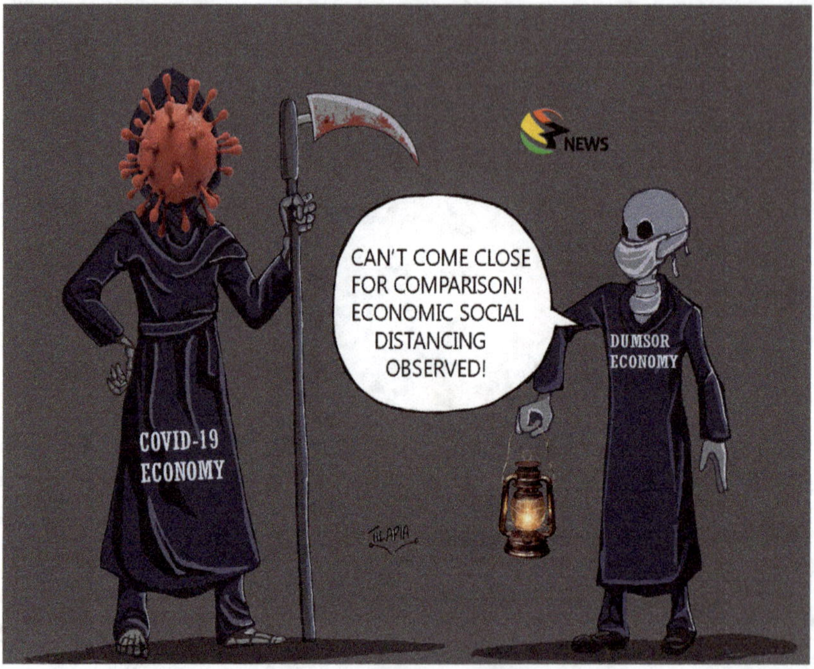
NEWS
CAN'T COME CLOSE FOR COMPARISON! ECONOMIC SOCIAL DISTANCING OBSERVED!
COVID-19 ECONOMY
DUMSOR ECONOMY
TILAPIA

Figure 8.11 'Dumsor-COVID-19 economy comparison', cartoon by Tilapia da Cartoonist 7 May 2020.

speculations and conspiracy theories circulating on social media, and in particular African Twitter, about the source of the pandemic and anti-African vaccine developments.

"Yɛte hɔ aa mo se Bird Flu (bird flu)	At first you all said Bird Flu (bird flu)
Ankyɛ na mo se Swine Flu (swine flu)	Soon after you said Swine Flu (swine flu)
Yɛbɛ te y'ɛni aa rabies (rabies)	Before we knew it was rabies (rabies)
Yɛda ne yɛn ho HIV (mokoraa adɛn!)	We turned around, HIV (what is it with you all!)
Afei na corona (rona)	Right now it is corona (rona)
Saa na mo yɛɛ Ebola (bola)	Same way you made Ebola (bola)

White man always tryna find ways
to eradicate black population
Oh no
Leave the Black alone"

On the surface, Tulenkey's song fed into infodemics – the blend of misinformation and disinformation on COVID-19 that had circulated on social media since January 2020 (Zarocostas, 2020). At a deeper level, it was a song that revealed the psychopolitics of the COVID-19 response. Tulenkey placed the Ghanaian story within the broader African context with his references to White versus Black people. He bemoaned Western interference in the lives of Africans: 'Oh no, leave the Black alone'. The song instantiated W. E. B. Du Bois's ([1903] 1965) concept of double consciousness – a mode of looking at Ghanaian and Black African realities through the lens of Western and White power structures. To understand how a Hiplife song could carry these psychopolitical elements, we have to examine the roots of African Twitter (now X) anxiety and simmering rage about perceived Western scientific experimentations on African populations.

The discourse on Africa in global health and politics took a predictable stigmatising path after the first cases of COVID-19 infections were reported on the continent. In April 2020, two senior French medics were talking on a French television network about the possible use of the BCG tuberculosis vaccine to treat COVID-19. One observed casually:

> If I could be provocative [. . .] Should we not do this study in Africa, where there are no [face] masks, no treatments and no ICUs? A bit like it is done for some studies on AIDS, where with prostitutes, we try things because we know that they are highly exposed and they don't protect themselves?[16]

The other agreed. The reaction on African Twitter (X) was swift. The WHO's director general, Dr Tedros Adhanom Ghebreyesus, publicly rebuked the medics, calling their remarks "racist" and a "hangover from a colonial mentality."[17]

As death rates rose in Europe and North America, the narrative of Africa as the world's laboratory for COVID-19 vaccine development shifted to a narrative of Africa as the world's imminent COVID-19 grave. Global health experts predicted catastrophic mortality rates in Africa – with estimates ranging from 300,000 to 3.3 million deaths (UN ECA, 2020). In an interview on CNN, the billionaire philanthropist Melinda French Gates remarked: "Look at Ecuador. They are putting bodies out on the street. You're going to see that in countries in Africa."[18] When these predictions failed, "the African COVID-19 paradox" was coined. One group of US-based epidemiologists defined the idea as follows: "Despite *its* crowded social life and poor personal hygiene practices, case fatality of

[16] "The two doctors appeared on French TV network LCI. The drug in question was undergoing clinical trials for that purpose in the Netherlands and Australia.

[17] Shaban (2020).

[18] Melinda Gates: This is what keeps me up at night – YouTube. Talking to Poppy Harlow on CNN, 10 April 2020.

COVID-19 has been paradoxically low in Africa compared to the Western world" (Ghosh et al., 2020, p.1, emphasis added).

In November 2021, when South African scientists alerted the world to the Omicron variant, a travel ban was imposed on eight southern African countries by the European Union, United Kingdom and United States. A German newspaper, Die Rheinpfalz, declared in a front-page headline: "The Virus from Africa Is with Us" (Das Virus aus Afrika ist bei uns). A Spanish newspaper, Tribuna de Albacete, published a cartoon depicting "Omicron variants as caricatured Black South Africans crammed in a boat heading for Europe".[19]

These ideas about Africans being carriers of the COVID-19 virus, when the pandemic originated in China and took its greatest toll in North America and Europe, clearly demonstrated the persistence of the trope of 'Africa as an infectious continent' in the global imagination. These global representations filtered through to continental and diaspora African communities in real-time via traditional and social media and fuelled engaged, and often outraged, discussions in these spaces. Tulenkey's song captured these psychopolitical themes.

Pandemic Arts and the Psychopolitics of COVID-19

Research on pandemic arts – from cholera outbreaks in nineteenth-century Britain and the 1918 Spanish flu in the United States to HIV/AIDS and Ebola in African countries since the 1980s – suggests that these art forms, whether they originate in spontaneous social responses or formal artistic productions, perform important public health functions (Barz and Cohen, 2011; Foss, 2020; Park and Park, 2010; Sonke and Pesata, 2015). Pandemic arts reduce social anxiety, tension and fear and offer 'hope and resilience' particularly for poor and marginalised communities (Barz and Cohen, 2011; Sonke and Pesata, 2015). Through the emotional connections they create, the arts also educate in ways that are more socially accessible, acceptable and engaging compared to formal public health approaches. Jill Sonke and Virginia Pesata (2015), writing on the impact of stories from Ebola survivors in Liberia, Sierra Leone and Guinea, observed that "when people engage emotionally with *correct information*

[19] See Greenhalgh and de-Graft Aikins (2023). The cartoon can be viewed in a blog by another cartoonist who was critical of its racist stereotyping: Anuncios. *The newspaper La Tribuna de Albacete and its cartoonist apologise for a cartoon*, published 1 December 2021 and accessed 30 June 2022: https://jrmora.com/en/the-newspaper-la-tribuna-de-albacete-cartoonist-apologise-cartoon/.

through the arts, they share that information with others, creating an organic and meaningful dissemination of knowledge" (p.6, emphasis added).

COVID arts operated through these socio-psychological mechanisms. Comedy, for example, helped people cope with the stresses of infection, caregiving and bereavement as the pandemic progressed. Channelling official prevention information through comedy also created deeper emotional connections with audiences and set the foundation for public understanding of a complex pandemic. As Barz and Cohen (2011) noted of HIV/AIDS messaging in Uganda, when audiences nodded their heads in agreement or clapped their hands in laughter to localised terminologies of AIDS that resonated with their lived experiences, they were much less threatened and anxious about the messages.

It is important to note that there were limitations to the communication functions of COVID arts. Some art forms provided correct scientific information that was disengaged from social contexts. State-sponsored arts such as the GGC and Hamid Nii Nortey murals, which focused solely on providing correct information, excluded important commentary on water poverty in many parts of the country, the prohibitive cost of disposable masks and hand sanitisers, and the cultural drivers of vaccination hesitancy. Other art forms projected mixed messages. Tulenkey's Hiplife song channelled conspiracy theories about the origins of COVID-19 that were rooted in collective memories and rational fears driven by historical biomedical injustices. But the song's message also contributed to shaping health-disabling attitudes around prevention and vaccination. Although Ghana was the first African country to receive vaccines in March 2021, vaccination rates remain low, partly because of vaccine distribution inequities and poor distribution nationally but also due to vaccination hesitancy. Although the WHO declared the end of the pandemic in May 2023, new waves continue to emerge, such as the wave in August 2023 driven by the 'Eris' or EG.5 variant (Tétrault-Farber and Leo, 2023). Prevention and vaccination remain important public health tasks.

Throughout the COVID-19 pandemic, there have been calls to re-imagine, restructure and redesign health systems to meet the complex demands of current and future global health threats (e.g., Assefa et al., 2021). This call is not new. The Millennium Development Goals (MDGs), adopted in 2000, ushered in the era of re-imagining health systems. The Sustainable Development Goals (SDGs) that followed in 2015 offered clear guidelines on addressing intersectional inequalities and forging global solidarity, which should have prepared the world for a multilayered global health crisis like COVID-19. But, as previous chapters have shown, the global health imagination is framed by a distorted Western gaze and a limited set of scientific disciplines, and it tends to exclude social imaginaries and social creativity – what ordinary people imagine, see, feel and want to create for themselves.

The idea of 'the African COVID paradox', for example, did not take into account the ways in which lived experiences of epidemiological complexity forge social creativity and resilience in African communities. For countries like Ghana that had experienced serial public health threats over decades, COVID-19 was a familiar alien threat: public understanding of its roots and impact was shaped by a deep collective knowledge of sickness, debility and death. Lay representations were cognitive polyphasic. Communities made sense of the pandemic by drawing simultaneously from medical science, ethnomedicine, religion, politics, culture and common sense – and worked through complex social emotions including amusement, fear, scepticism, anger and hope. In Ghana and elsewhere, there was also concrete action: lay communities, scientific communities, religious institutions and private sector companies developed homegrown prevention and treatment solutions (Eribo, 2021). These responses mimicked lay African responses to HIV/AIDS in the early years of the crisis (see Chapter 1).

Local artists working across genres translated these scientific, socio-cultural and political trends. A radical subset – who fit the description, provided by Karin Barber (1987, p.1), of artists that "flourish without encouragement or recognition from official cultural bodies, and sometimes in defiance of them" – exposed the coloniality of Ghana's official health system by making deeper connections between history, politics and policy. For example, the localised term 'colonial virus' started as an inside cultural joke – one of several lay mispronunciations of 'coronavirus' that went viral on social media in March 2020 (this one of 'Twinglish'). Then artists like Clemento Suarez, Tilapia da Cartoonist and Tulenkey reworked the joke through comedy, cartoons and songs as a critique of the 'colonial mentality' driving inequitable political responses to the COVID-19 pandemic and to previous pandemics such as Ebola, swine flu and HIV/AIDS. Their artistic stance and messaging had a conscientising force. These artists, as Barber (1987) observed of the power of 'truly popular art', opened the eyes of their vast audiences to the objective reality of health inequalities and primed them to take collective action.

CHAPTER 9

Conclusions

In Ghana here, you have to be creative to move ahead
Benjamin Aidoo, Head of Nana Otafirija Pallbearing and Waiting Service, 2017

Globally and in African settings, the arts have been integrated into health promotion, disease prevention, illness management and policy development. This integration has occurred in a number of ways. The arts have been used to explore local experiences and understandings of health, to fashion health education messages, to provide therapy for a range of conditions and to evaluate, validate and disseminate health research findings.

In Ghana, the arts have been applied to official and semi-official health communication projects since the establishment of formal biomedical services in the colonial era. Official projects are those implemented and/or funded by government and their donor and collaborative partners; semi-official projects are those conceptualised and implemented by researchers with formal institutional affiliations, with or without official funding. Interventions employing film, television drama, theatre, songs, stories, slogans, recipes and art exhibitions have sought to educate communities on disease prevention (e.g., syphilis, cholera, HIV, NCDs) and disease stigma reduction (e.g., HIV, mental illness), and, for a limited number of projects, to improve illness management (e.g., mental illness and NCDs) and general well-being (e.g., eating healthily). The arts have also been used as research tools, such as the use of theatre to examine youth representations of HIV/AIDS and photovoice to examine community perspectives on nutrition risks.

These interventions have co-existed, often in real time, with creative responses to a wider set of health threats in lay communities and the use of the arts within indigenous healing systems. Lay communities and local artists have responded to pandemic health threats such as HIV/AIDS and COVID-19, for instance, by drawing on long-standing arts traditions such as musical performance, satire, funerary arts and textile arts. Indigenous healers have always carved out a powerful niche in the pluralistic healthcare system through the multi-form arts they activate, from the use of wall art for advertising services to the use of medical devices as performative healing objects.

The arts and health field in Ghana has not developed to the extent that research has been conducted and evaluated across all the healthcare domains, for a wide range of health conditions, using the common integration approaches.

For example, research has demonstrated the impact of singing on well-being and building social bonds, via the subjective accounts of people living with mental illness or lay people listening to and singing along to AIDS songs. However, there has been no exploration of the physiological and physical impact of singing. Downes and colleagues (2019) examined the impact of singing on secondary prevention of chronic respiratory disease in an outpatient clinic in Kampala, Uganda. They observed that "many of the muscles required for posture and breathing control are the same used when singing" (p.220). These cardiorespiratory and muscular demands constituted a form of physical activity that improved symptoms for chronic obstructive pulmonary disorders and lung obstruction problems. When patients and healthcare providers sang together, they reported improved interpersonal relationships in the clinical environment. Singing also offered a cheaper, more enjoyable physical activity option for patients that could be added to evidence-based illness management guidelines for chronic respiratory illness.

A second limitation is that the dominant focus of interventions has been on adult populations. In the supplementary scoping review of seventeen arts-based health studies conducted between the late 1980s and 2020 (see Appendix 1), only two peer-reviewed studies focused on children and young people: a malaria prevention project using the Ananse story to create prevention messages (Gotfried, 2014) and a dance drama project on malaria and cholera prevention that involved school-age children as peer educators (Frishkopf et al., 2016, see The Arts and Health Communication Ecosystem in Ghana). We saw in Chapter 4 youth choirs creating and singing AIDS songs, young people communicating their knowledge of HIV/AIDS risk through participatory theatre, and singing children alerting community members in Konko to new AIDS songs. In these case studies, the value of children and youth as co-creators of health communication was evident. In lay communities, the value of children as communicators of popular ideas is understood. Mempeasem President's sketch on herbal centres, presented in Chapter 2, included a popular phrase that captures this shared understanding: "When you ask even a child, about Kpomegbe Herbal Center, you will be directed to our centre." Traditional and social media reports highlight the way schools harness this value in arts education. Elite schools with art departments and programmes facilitate creative student projects and events for 'their schools' and wider communities – such as plays and concerts performed at the National Theatre in Accra. Schools with fewer resources collaborate with local arts organisations, who co-produce arts-based activities with children. In the entertainment world, television programmes like TV3's *Talented Kids* showcase the creative abilities of child contestants representing all the regions of the country. More work needs to be done to synthesise the insights from these activities to inform child- and youth-centred health communication interventions.

Finally, while there is strong evidence of the cost-effectiveness of arts-based interventions compared to usual public health interventions in Global North settings (see for example Fancourt and Finn, 2019), definitive statements cannot be made about cost-effectiveness in the Ghanaian context as few arts-based health interventions have been costed. In the scoping review, only one project provided details on costs. Canadian ethnomusicologist Michael Frishkopf and colleagues (2016) applied dance drama to malaria and cholera education in four communities – Gbungbalaga, Jekeriyili (Tamale), Tolon, Ziong – in the Northern Region. The project cost CAD 5000.00 per community performance. The amount covered compensation to professional artists ('for whom music is a livelihood'), transportation, roadies who assembled and disassembled the stage and operated the sound system, and traditional protocols (such as presenting drinks to chiefs and traditional leaders). Frishkopf and colleagues observed that while they "compensated all participants fairly, it was impossible to imagine how [they] could raise the funds needed to provide such continuity, since the total cost would linearly increase over time" (p.63).

However, by focusing on health communication and existing evaluation of selected projects in this domain, the functions and impact of the arts for health promotion and disease prevention are captured, and we are also afforded glimpses of what the arts can do for illness management and for health policy. And by examining the "creative resources people bring to their own healing" (Philips et al., 2020), we see the intersecting "aesthetic, spiritual, social" (Cole and Ross, 1977), as well as psychological and political dynamics underpinning health communication in these domains. Four cross-cutting insights emerge from the featured case studies.

First, the case studies underscore the value of the arts as a medium for health promotion and disease prevention. Songs communicate health themes in powerful ways across communities, for all age groups, especially when they are used in nationwide mass media campaigns. In some cases, the impact of songs lasts long after the intervention for which they were produced. For example, *Hohorowonsa*, the song created for The Truly Clean Hands campaign in 2003, served a new purpose during the first year of COVID-19 for musicians and comedians creating COVID-19 messaging for a new audience. Lay communities suggest that songs operate at cognitive, emotional and physical levels: they work when they have pleasing, memorable melodies – simple enough for children to sing – danceable rhythms, are sung clearly in local languages and contain sound, applicable advice.

Theatre works when storylines clearly delineate target health problems and when they reflect the life experiences of audience members. For some members of participating communities, there is a preference for indigenous forms of theatre, like the concert party, that are performed in local languages and incorporate other participatory arts such as comedy, singing and dancing. For performers, theatre can lessen anxieties about disclosing difficult personal stories and taboo subjects. When storytelling – through community theatre or television drama – strikes a cultural chord for the general population or for subgroups, such as with *Things We Do for Love*, its impact can last beyond the life of the project for which it was developed, through the activation of social memory and nostalgia.

Visual arts, from billboard images of HIV/AIDS to paintings and photographs on mental health themes, forge cognitive and emotional connections to the target health issues. People remember the emaciated HIV/AIDS sufferer because they have seen imagery on billboards, television adverts and other multimedia campaign paraphernalia. For visitors to a mental health exhibition, photographs of individuals with mental illness in indigenous healing settings introduce a new way of seeing the impact of mental illness on families that is visceral and therefore memorable. The key lies in the social psychological phenomenon of objectification – where the unfamiliar or familiar alien threats are reproduced "among the things we can see and touch and thus control" (Moscovici, 1984, p.29) giving novelty or the uncanny a "concrete, almost natural face" (Jovchelovitch, 2001, p.172).

Satire, comedy sketches, cartoons and funerary arts provide an entry point into 'creative practices of the imagination' within the context of public health threats. These art forms illustrate how humour operates at the social level, for lay people and artists: to facilitate the communication of complex health information (such as comedy, cartoons and funerary arts for COVID-19), to criticise and hold powerful institutions accountable (such as satirical sketches on fake herbalists and pastors) and to cope with unsettling new public health threats.

Secondly, the case studies demonstrate that the arts, like all expressive forms, have limits and unintended consequences. These dynamics must be understood in the development of interventions. There are limitations to the use of arts in edutainment. Communities warn that there has to be a careful balance between entertaining and educating: "if the music is too beautiful, it makes you shake to the beat instead of listening to the words" as a community member in the Eastern Region remarked (Bosompra, 2007–2008, p.146). Telling personal stories of illness can lead to or intensify stigma.

New images can cause symbolic harm. Early HIV/AIDS campaigns introduced "transnational imagescapes" (Quayson, 2014) of the disease that joined other images circulating in the symbolic social environment and in social imaginaries, became a subject of communication, a constituent of social practices, and the (re)construction of reality. This objectification process reshaped ideas about serious sickness, perpetuated pre-existing stereotypes in society and deepened stigmatising practices that persist today.

There are limits to creativity and innovation in indigenous healing spaces. These limits emerge through the discrepancy between the performance of healing – from the use of representations of small gods in shrines to spectacular machines in modern herbal clinics – and concrete health outcomes. The harmful side of creativity in indigenous healing systems is unmasked and challenged through lay stories and satire, illustrating that healing systems are subjected to social scrutiny and critique, and secondly that these communicative processes are undergirded by social creativity.

Thirdly, community-based participatory methods – which involve co-production, but also a relatively longer period of social engagement – facilitate a deeper understanding of community views on their prevalent health problems, which is crucial for mapping the social determinants of health and contextualising health interventions. In Konko and Koforidua, community members placed HIV/AIDS within the context of a broader infectious disease burden. Across RHN communities, there was a shared awareness of the impact of toxic agriculture and environmental degradation on the quality and safety of food. Here, the arts functioned as methods of data elicitation, as community health knowledge was examined within the context of reflections on the broader arts-based projects. The value of arts within mixed methods data elicitation designs has been reported for other projects, such as the dance drama project developed by Frishkopf and colleagues (2016) for malaria and cholera prevention in the Northern region.

Finally, while the three forms of arts-based health communication operate within an ecological system, there has been no sustained attempt – bar collaborations in mental healthcare – to integrate practices and lessons across expert and lay domains. This problem must be understood as an artefact of Ghana's official healthcare system within which health communication and health promotion projects are conceptualised and implemented.

The Arts and Health Communication Ecosystem in Ghana

The three forms of arts-based health communication operate within an ecological system that maps onto the Whole of Government, Whole of Society (WoG, WoS) model described in Chapter 7, and is illustrated in Figure 9.1 below.

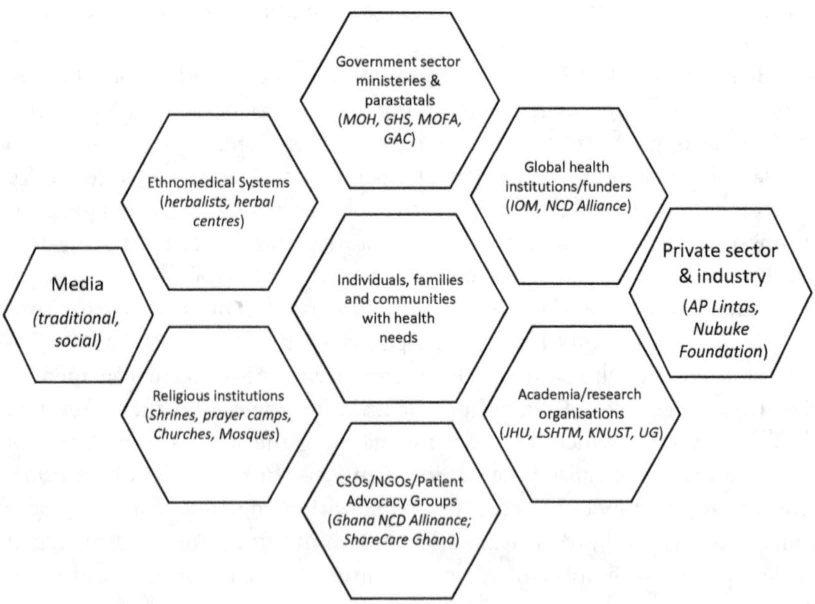

Figure 9.1 Arts and health communication ecosystem in Ghana.

From the WoG end, the relevant public service agencies include the Ministry of Health and Ghana Health Service, a selection of sector ministries (such as the Ministry of Food and Agriculture and Ministry of Fisheries and Aquaculture Development) and parastatals (such as the Ghana AIDS Commission), as well as institutional allies in the donor (e.g., USAID) and global health (e.g., NCD Alliance) sectors. From the WoS end, a heterogeneous set of social and institutional groups operate, including patient support groups, mass media, marketing and public relations firms, and cultural and arts foundations.

Generally, as we saw with NCD policy in Chapter 7, public service agencies do not "work across portfolio boundaries to develop integrated policies and programmes" (Ortenzi et al., 2022, p.1). Furthermore, health communication is largely anti-dialogical, so there is a lack of integration with stakeholders that make up the WoS domain. Within the WoS domain itself, there is heterogeneity in the way arts are created, engaged with and used for health communication. Patient support groups deploy life stories to advocate for health conditions. Mass media promotes conflicting health messages from pluralistic health systems. Marketing firms provide creative expertise on health communication interventions, but (are forced to) do so in ways that ignore complex social realities. Cultural and arts foundations support local arts groups in ad hoc and siloed ways.

The 'anti-dialogical banking education' approach that dominates health communication models and projects drives a deeper conceptual wedge between expert and lay communicative domains. While arts lie at the heart of lay communication, the arts are treated as an add-on feature in expert-led health communication projects. For example, when AIDS songs or RHN slogans or COVID-19 murals and official songs were developed, these art forms were incorporated superficially – and the broader messages were decontextualised from complex social realities. The songs were informed by fear appeals which ignored or underestimated shifting cultural representations of good death and bad death and the complex socio-psychological dimensions of fear. The RHN slogans promoted messages that ignored the social psychological impact of 'slow observations' of the slow violence of environmental degradation on food cultures and the double burden of malnutrition. The COVID-19 murals and songs presented sanitised images and narratives of prevention that did not take into account disabling factors like water poverty and unequal access to health goods. And, as we saw with the Truly Clean Hands campaign in Chapter 3, where local partners were employed as part of the know-nothing receiving communities, the conceptual role of artists in official projects was often unclear.

There is a consensus within the arts and health field in Africa that when government or funding agency projects employ anti-dialogical banking education approaches, a "communicative deadlock" rooted in fixed expectations from both sides ensues: "shared meaning scarcely emerges between the parties" (Beck, 2006, p.537). This communicative deadlock is a core feature of the psychopolitics of encounters between experts and lay communities. In many cases, as we saw for colonial projects such as the mothercraft project in colonial Asante, and more recent global health interventions for HIV/AIDS, NCDs and COVID-19, the anti-dialogical approach is resisted or reworked to serve local purposes. What is required in African settings, as several theorists have argued, is a dialogical and people-centred approach to health communication, whether projects apply mass-media campaigns or community-based participatory methods. The dominant approach whereby local people participate in experts' projects must give way to experts participating in the projects of local people (Chinyowa, 2015). By turning the lens onto the creative resources ordinary people bring to their own representations of, and practical responses to, health, illness and healing, experts can fashion more robust dialogical, people-centred health communication models.

To move from theory to practice will require a community of practice: "a group created over time by the sustained pursuit of a shared enterprise, bound by mutual engagements, shared cultural practices and common social commitments" (Frishkopf et al., 2016, p.49, citing Wenger, 1998). Within the arts and health communication ecosystem, and in the areas of mental healthcare particularly, there are important overlaps across the activities of a subset of lay community groups, indigenous healers, patient groups, multidisciplinary researchers, artists, art foundations, healthcare providers and funders. This offers a familiar collaborative and pragmatic testing ground to develop and implement transformational arts-based health communication models.

But like participatory health projects everywhere, arts-based health interventions that aim to transform the health and well-being of participating groups and sustain impact in the long term, require substantial financial support as well as local ownership (Campbell et al., 2007; Cornish et al., 2023; Frishkopf et al., 2016). As Frishkopf and colleagues (2016, p.63) observed of their dance drama project on malaria and cholera prevention in Northern Ghana:

> the problem concerned more than just financial sustainability; it concerned also social sustainability through local engagement. We posed as a PAR (participatory action research) project, but with what level of participation?

> Community participation is crucial not only to guide a project, but to ensure its long-term viability, because in supporting itself, the community acts out self-interest, and naturally adapts to changing conditions.

Sankofa: Indigenising Health Communication

When Benjamin Aidoo observes that 'in Ghana you have to be creative to move ahead', he speaks of the hustle/galamsey[1] culture that shapes new modes of economic production for pastors, healers, serial entrepreneurs and creatives. In essence, he draws attention to how a Kwaku Bonsam, Nana Agraada or a herbal centre CEO is created, or how fellow local artists like Clemento Suarez and Tilapia da Cartoonist flourish despite severely limited government support for the arts. His observation can also be applied to the creativity required for an ordinary individual to find health-care solutions in a health marketplace that can be inaccessible, expensive and harmful, as we saw for Aba and her mother in Mullings' (1984) study, or for Solo and Mama in Yankah's (2004) study.

In developing people-centred dialogical health communication models to serve individuals and communities with complex health needs, much can be learned from creative strategies employed by indigenous healers and lay communities. To further this argument, I use the concept of Sankofa as an organising principle for reclaiming arts traditions for official health communication. In Chapter 1, I defined Sankofa as 'a creative practice of the imagination and memory – a vital process of remembering and reclaiming lost or contested traditions within the boundaries of self, society and culture and activating these traditions to serve contemporary needs'.

The Sankofa principle has always informed the workings of indigenous healers. Like the proverbial Sankofa bird that moves forward while its head is turned backwards, the reinvention of healing traditions requires that healers look back as they move forward. They borrow strategically from eclectic sources to modernise their services even as they protect the core functions of indigenous healing: that is to address the interactions between the physical and spiritual dimensions of serious sickness. The arts are utilised as a knowledge system in diagnosing and healing. Representations of small gods, everyday objects loaded with spiritual power, small medical objects and spectacular machines aid the

[1] Coined from the English phrase 'gather and sell', galamsey is a subversive practice that emerged in response to discriminatory colonial policies that rendered traditional artisanal mining illegal, to pave way for mining by the colonial state and big-money foreign interests (Addo-Fening, 2013). The term is still used for prohibited mining activities, but it has also become a catch-all term for all kinds of creative and subversive money-making schemes.

performance of diagnosis and treatment. And if spiritual imaginaries – which bridge the visible and invisible worlds – are aligned between healers and clients, and shared belief is strong, the performances become channels for healing, whether symbolic or concrete.

The Sankofa principle also informs the use of arts in social life. To illustrate this point, we must revisit the major life events outlined in the introductory chapter for which arts play central roles: out-doorings, puberty rites, marriage ceremonies and funerals. These family and community events operate in similar ways to the festival (as 'art event'), in the sense that "time, people and scale lift ordinary and ritualised activities into the realm of art" (Cole and Ross, 1977). At each event, there is collective reflection of the power of the past weighing in on the present when ancestors are called through libation and the verbal arts (proverbs, retelling of clan stories) that mediate this process; when formal speeches are enhanced with song and dance, when bodies are adorned with commissioned textiles or beads handed down through generations; when family and gendered roles and functions are delineated through carefully curated colour schemes; when specific cuisines are prescribed and consumed. At these events, art is truly participatory. To paraphrase Suzanne Preston Blier (1993, p.147) there is a 'complex interweave of individuals who both participate in the creative process as artists' – musicians, singers, dancers, fashion designers, linguists – 'and bring signification to the work through their divergent roles' as hosts, guests, or subjects for which the events have been convened. Art also functions politically: individuals can subvert family and community norms and power dynamics for personal and group social capital. Funerals bring this element to the fore most vividly (see Appiah, 1992). The art forms themselves change over time – new elements are borrowed and meanings and forms of engagement change with evolving social, economic and political conditions. When activated positively, these arts-based rituals mediate social connections and cultural renewal and push families and social groups into new relational spaces. They create pleasure, joy and other positive social emotions that enhance well-being in specific moments and across time through shared memories.

It is this intermingling of the aesthetic, spiritual, social, psychological and political in healing and social spaces that make arts and social creativity powerful mediating forces for transformational health communication. And in the same way that radical artists "flourish independently of official cultural bodies, and sometimes in defiance of them" (Barber, 1987, p.1), lay communities will continue to produce health their way with or without official interventions. The evolution of healing environments will follow suit.

APPENDIX I

Map Showing Sites of Arts-Based Interventions

Map of Ghana Showing Sites of Arts-based Health Interventions

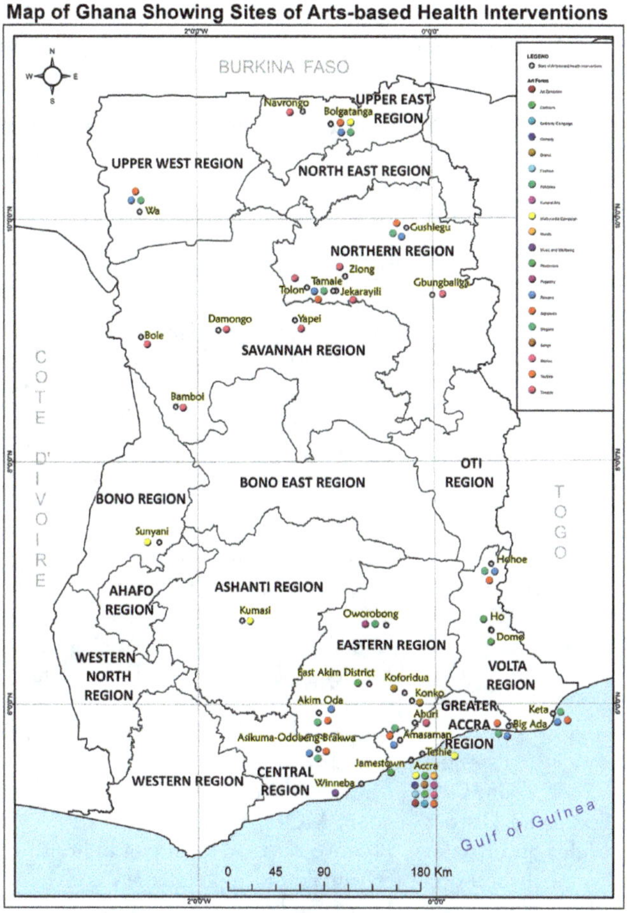

Note on Studies and Study Locations

A scoping review of arts-based health studies was conducted to map the arts and health field in Ghana, as presented above in the Map of Ghana Showing Sites of Arts-based Health Interventions (see also de-Graft Aikins et al, 2024). This table presents brief descriptions of the seventeen identified studies, which were conducted between the late 1980s and 2020. Studies were included in the review if they: (1) used art forms as a research method and/or intervention; (2) focused on a health condition or risk factor; and (3) provided descriptions of the art-based methods, however brief. A selection of these studies are featured as case studies in Chapters 3, 4, 6 and 8.

Regions (towns, communities)	Studies (art-based health interventions)
Ashanti Region Kumasi Unspecified town/community	Multi-media campaign (a magazine, movies, a radio program, song, social media): smoking prevention (Hutchinson et al., 2020) Pictorial warning labels: smoking prevention (Singh et al., 2014) Multi-media campaign (television and radio adverts using a slogan and song, billboards, stickers): handwashing (Scott et al., 2008) Multi-media campaign (billboards, song, videos, leaflets): HIV/AIDS stigma (Boulay et al., 2008)
Brong Ahafo Region Sunyani	Multi-media campaign: smoking prevention (Hutchinson et al., 2020)
Central Region Asikuma-Odobeng-Brakwa Winneba	Multi-media campaign (slogans, signposts, celebrity campaign): regenerative health and nutrition (RHN) (de-Graft Aikins, 2010; MOH, 2012) Choral singing: general well-being (Acquah, 2016) Music: general health and well-being (Carl, 2016)
Eastern Region Aburi Akim-Oda East Akim District Koforidua and Konko Oworobong	Theatre and HIV/AIDS prevention (Boneh and Jaganath, 2011) Multi-media campaign: RHN (de-Graft Aikins, 2010; MOH, 2012) Photovoice: food security and health (Nyantakyi-Frimpong et al., 2021) Drama and HIV/AIDS education (Bosompra, 2007–2008) Puppetry and Ananse stories: malaria education (Gotfried, 2014)

Location	Study
Greater Accra Region East Legon, Pantang, Accra Amasaman, Big Ada Jamestown, Accra Korle-Bu, Accra Teshie, Accra Unspecified, Accra	Art exhibition: mental health promotion (de-Graft Aikins, 2009) Multi-media campaign: RHN (de-Graft Aikins, 2010; MOH, 2012) Photovoice: food security and health (Pradeilles et al., 2021) Stories/narratives: HIV/AIDS experiences (Yankah, 2004) Multi-media campaign: smoking behaviour (Hutchinson et al., 2020) Multi-media, 'grandmother tales': general health (Ansu-Kyeremeh et al., 2016) Multi-form arts (cartoons; comedy; murals; music; textiles): COVID-19 (de-Graft Aikins and Akoi-Jackson, 2020)
Northern and Savannah Regions Bamboi, Bole, Damongo, Navrongo, Yapei Gbungbalaga, Jekeriyili (Tamale), Tolon, Ziong Tamale, Gushegu	Theatre: HIV/AIDS prevention (Boneh and Jaganath, 2011) Dance drama: malaria and cholera (Frishkopf, Hamze, et al, 2016; Frishkopf et al., 2016) Multi-media campaign: RHN (de-Graft Aikins, 2010; MOH, 2012)
Upper East Region Bolgantanga Unspecified town/community	Multi-media campaign: RHN (de-Graft Aikins, 2010; MOH, 2012) Multi-media campaign: hygiene behaviours (Scott et al., 2008)
Upper West Region Wa	Multi-media campaign: RHN (de-Graft Aikins, 2010; MOH, 2012)
Volta Region Domo, Ho Hohoe, Keta	Photovoice: food security and health (Pradeilles et al., 2021) Multi-media campaign: RHN (de-Graft Aikins, 2010; MOH, 2012)
Western Region Unspecified town/community	Multi-media campaign: hygiene behaviours (Scott et al., 2008)

APPENDIX 2

Interviews

Note: For the majority of the chapters, I have drawn on interviews and focus group discussions from previous research on chronic illness representations and experiences (e.g., de-Graft Aikins, 2005; de-Graft Aikins et al., 2020). But I also conducted, with a team, the following new individual, dyadic and group interviews that explored current Ghanaian trends in the arts and in arts and health. I present a list of interviewees, noting who conducted the interviews (full names first, followed by initials), the interview dates and locations:

1. Selected members of Act for Change, a Jamestown-based arts organisation, including Collins Seymah Smith and Hamid Nii Nortey. Group discussion and interviews facilitated by Ama de-Graft Aikins (AdGA), June 2019, Accra.
2. Dr Bernard Akoi-Jackson, artist and academic. Interview by AdGA, August 2019, Kumasi.
3. Professor Ablade Glover, artist, academic and owner of the Artists Alliance Gallery, Accra. Interview by AdGA and Grace Brew-Appiah, December 2020, Accra.
4. Mrs Frances Ademola, art patron and owner of the Loom Gallery, the first art gallery in Accra. Interview by AdGA, May 2021, Accra.
5. Ms Nana Yaa Agyeman, Founder of Sharecare Ghana. Interview by Dr Ernestina Tetteh, September 2021, Accra.
6. Christopher Agbeba, Advocacy Manager of Sharecare Ghana. Interviews by AdGA, October 2021, April 2023, Accra.
7. Fatric Bewong, artist. Interview by AdGA, December 2021, Accra.
8. Eric Kwakyi, advertising executive, formerly of Mullen Lowe Accra. Interview by AdGA, May 2022, Accra.
9. Barbara Davies, Executive Director and Yoofi Brew, Creative Director, Mullen Lowe Accra. Interview by AdGA, May 2022, Accra.

10. Dr Sela Adjei, artist and academic. Interviews by AdGA, May 2022, February 2023, Accra.
11. Tilapia da Cartoonist, artist. Interview by AdGA, September 2022, Accra.
12. Jamestown Children's Health Club. Group discussions facilitated by Vida Asah-Ayeh (VAA), 2022, Accra.
13. Jamestown Health Club. Group discussions facilitated by VAA, 2022, Accra.
14. Jeff Klein, artist and curator, Global Groove. Interview by AdGA, March 2023, New Orleans.
15. Labram Musah, National Coordinator of Ghana NCD Alliance. Interview by AdGA, April 2023, Accra.
16. Florence Okine, textiles trader. Interview by Jemima Okai (JO), May 2023, Accra.
17. Hamza Ibrahim, artist based at the Accra Arts Centre. Interview by JO, August 2023, Accra.
18. Nai Wulomo, Chief Priest of Ga Mashie. Interview by VAA, March 2024, Accra.
19. Leslie Mills Lamptey, aka Great Ozonkponu ("the saint"), Chief Priest's PRO. Interview by VAA, March 2024, Accra.

APPENDIX 3

Selected Primary and Secondary Data

APPENDIX 3A

Images

Ga Mashie Chief Priest's Mural (Recommissioned in 2020)

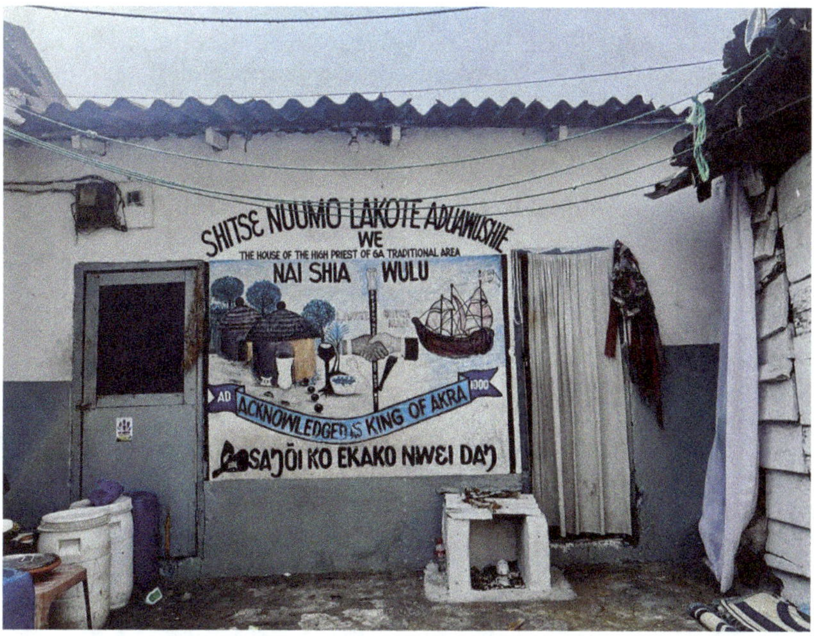
SHITSƐ NUUMO LAKOTE ADUAWUSHIE
WE
THE HOUSE OF THE HIGH PRIEST OF GA TRADITIONAL AREA
NAI SHIA WULU
AD
1000
ACKNOWLEDGED AS KING OF AKRA
SAŊÕI KO EKAKO NWƐI DAŊ

Photograph by Jemima Okai, March 2024.

Annotation of Added Visual Features

Information is based on an interview with the Chief Priest, Nai Wulomo (NW) conducted by Vida Asah-Ayeh (VAA) in March 2024.

[1] The four black pots leading to the first hut

NW: When someone comes here, that is what we use to serve water.

VAA: Okay. So, please, why have they been arranged in a line?

NW: So that people will be aware of such a thing here. You cannot keep things you do in secret.

[2] The white stool in front of the first hut

VAA: what the significance of the stool in front of the hut?

NW: That is what I am currently sitting on. It signifies that that is what we Wulome sit on. [. . .] We will only sit on a different chair if it becomes critical especially when we go to some other place. We cannot request they give us our special seat. [. . .] A long time ago, they used to take [the stool] along. But now, it is difficult to do that.

[3] The gankogui double gongs or agogo bells (bottom left)

VAA: We realized that the gong-gong was not included [in the previous mural] but it has been included in the new one.

NW: It has been included in the new one. It signifies that I do not dance to any ordinary tunes. I dance only to the gong-gong tune. That is what we beat. Sakumo people play drums and they have people who play it. But as for us, it is the gong-gong that represents our voice.

[Note: This is a typical case of strategic cultural borrowing, as the gankogui double gongs are historically associated with Ewe musical traditions.]

APPENDIX 3B.

Song Lyrics

Song Title: Stop AIDS, Love Life

Artists: Ghana All Stars (Shasha Marley, Tic Tac, Chicago, Friction (Formerly of VIP), Gyedu Blay Ambolley, Black Prophet, Stella Dugan (now known as Stella Aba Seal), Diana Akiwumi (now Hopeson), Reggie Rockstone, Cy Lover, Cecil Pesewa (NFL), Original Ras Kobby, The Sheperds, Felix Owusu & Daasebre Gyamena)
Source: Tina Suliman on Youtube (Published on 3 November 2011) – www.youtube.com/watch?v=RPKVmxeoY4k
Duration: 6 minutes, 20 seconds
Languages: English, Ewe, Ga, Hausa, Fante, Jamaican Patois, Pidgin English, Twi
Transcription: Jemima Okai, Ruth Anokye, Sadick Osman, Comfort Ameka
Translation: Jemima Okai, Ruth Anokye, Sadick Osman, Comfort Ameka and Ama de-Graft Aikins

Shasha Marley: Oh oh oh. Jah has sent me as a messenger to warn you about this HIV
Tic Tac: Peace my friend
Shasha Marley: Stand firm or you gonna fall/'f*** -up'.
Chorus (All Stars)

You can maintain one lover,
it's not on it's not in,
you can wait until marriage.
Love life, Stop AIDS.

Tic Tac (Twi)

Ohh choo. . . Tic Tac ma bɛ duru. Hwɛ na wanka ankyerɛ me sɛ wo hyɛ 'rɔba' no wo ho baa ntɛm. Yaa Ataa, yɛ na kɔ hu dorkota no ntɛm. Me nbra biom? Me ngyae mmarimasɛm? ɛnnɛ metumi abɛ tena wo dan mu ntɛm. Me ne wo a, anka m'ɛsan ooo. Mɛ hye biom na madi me ho dɛm. Tic Tac, ɛyɛ ampa. Amanfoɔ, monhwɛ me o. Yareɛ bɔ wo a, ɔfe wɔɔwɔɔ, ne ti pae no o. Pɔmpɔ bɔ n'amotuom. Mɛyɛ no dɛn na m'atena fie. Memma dan mu ooo.

Ohh choo (sound of brakes) . . .Tic Tac, I've arrived. Do not tell me the rubber(condom) got torn whilst wearing it because you ejaculated early. Yaa Ataa, let us quickly visit the doctor. Should I come again? Should I stop having sex with multiple partners? Then I can quickly come to your room. If I were you, I retreat. I'd wear the condom again to be safe. Tic Tac, it's true. People, look at me. The symptoms of AIDS include vomiting, headache, boils. I can't stay home. I can't be inside.

Chicago (Ewe)

Mega Woe mewoge, dole yea AIDS Leoge, nemenga wowoe ekukuge. Enye Chicago ele nyae demdego. Nemedi yeakpor dolelee yea la. Lor amedeka alo n'aza nuyi woyaxe be condom-la, nakper nutifafa. Ne mea dukor nanor dziyim. Kabakaba tsoo kabakaba

Do not do it, I will do it, this sickness it is called AIDS. If you do not know, it will kill you. I am Chicago, I am telling if you do not want this disease, then love only one person or have only one partner. Use what we call condom, so you run away from this disease. So that there will be progress or peace in our nation. Fast fast ..

Friction VIP (Hausa)

Maata da ku muke, za muyimuku gargadi da wanan mugun chiwo HIV ke kachewa. Da baba, da mma, walahi kun ji ko. Wanan chiwo HIV walahi bashi da kaw. Wanan gargadi Friction ya rawaito. Ko kaki, ko kaso walahi munfada.

Ladies, we are here to advice you about the deadly HIV/AIDS disease that kills people. To the fathers, mothers, you should know that HIV is a bad disease. Friction is the one sending this message across. Whether you accept or decline the message, we have done our part by enlightening you.

Shasha Marley: It is real my brethren
All: You can maintain one lover.
Shasha Marley: Rastafari has come to warn you
All: it's not on, it's not in
Shasha Marley: What a killer disease
All: You can wait until marriage.
Shasha Marley: They got no remedy
All: Love life, Stop AIDS.

Gyedu Blay Amboley (Fante & English)

Se ɛhu sɛnea ewiade kɔ de yie, sɛ wo ahu die me kyere de yia, its all about

See how the world is going my dear, I'm pleading with you when you go

AIDS. Don't forget your condom, what they call rubber socks, ɔno na wɔfre no condom.

out it's all about AIDS. Don't forget your condom, what they call rubber socks.

Stella Dugan (Fante)

Dzi no kware kyerɛ wohokafo. Sɛ etwitwa akyiri aa wo bo ho dɛ bɔne ensuma da oo. AIDS yareba, sɛ ɛbɛ kɔ'aba fie aa, na wereho aba ooo

Be faithful to your partner. If anything, let them know. Don't send AIDS home to bring sadness.

Diana Akiwumi (Twi)

Nti dɔ wo nyanko, sɛ wo ho sɛ wodɔ wo nyako aa, wo nyɛ no bɔne da oo. Ma Nyame ndi woannim wo akwan nyinaa mu, na asomdwee bɛ ba oo

So, love your neighbor as yourself. If you love your neighbor, you will never sin against them. Let God lead you in all your ways and peace will reign.

Shasha Marley: ooh ooh ooh
All: You can maintain one lover.
Shasha Marley: Rastafari ee
All: it's not on, it's not in
Shasha Marley: It is a killer (x3)
All: You can wait until marriage.
Shasha Marley: Can't stop knowing
All: Love life, Stop Aids.
Shasha Marley: Oh mama hear my cry

Reggie Rockstone [00:03:26] [Twi]

Ah ɛnye ndra yi aa na me ne Kwamena ɛte ha edi nkɔmɔ yi, ende mekɔ bisaa na se aa yɛse ɔkɔ. . . Question? De ben na ɛyɛ no aa mo nyinaa mo ayɛ koom. Answer? Yareɛ keseɛ na ne dindin ketekete akyeno ama wawu. ɔde no kɔ ɔmba biom. Wo ngyedi aa diale www.nsamanpom .com. Wo hye shoe aa, hye socks na ewiase mu ayɛ huhuuhu. Wo te Accra wo tumi nya puncher.

Wasn't it just yesterday that Kwamena and I were chatting? I asked about him today and they said he's gone. Question, what happened to him that you've all been silent? Answer, that big disease with a small name took him away. He's gone and he's not coming back. If you don't believe me dial www.ghostworld.com. When you wear your shoes, wear socks because the world has become dangerous.

Cy Lover

Charley there's nothing wrong with having good sex but use a condom, there are many to select; Secure, Cutters and you can do it right. Use your condom chale and protect your health.

Cecil Pesewa (Pidgin)

AIDS be real, bɛ yo sabi the deal. The last girl wey you chop can be your last meal.

AIDS is real you understand the deal, the last girl you sleep with can be your last meal.

Original Ras Kobby

We're telling you AIDS(x3) is a dangerous disease. I'm advising. AIDS(x3), a conditional disease. I'm warning. Put on your condom, protect this kingdom. Protection before the action. Attention prevent abortion. Original Ras Kobby warning

The Shepherds (Ga)

Kɛ awie ni onuuɛ, onaa kɛ ohiŋmɛi. AIDS tamɔ la ni miɔɔ mɔ ja gbele, kɛ ohe aka ha lɛ kraa ni efite bo. Shi ohe hia kɛ ha Ghana maŋ mu fɛɛɛ.

When we speak and you don't listen, you will see with your eyes. AIDS is like fire until you die from it, don't give yourself the chance to be damaged by it, because you are important to Ghana.

Felix Owusu (Fante)

Muma yɛ hwɛ ni yie oo, AIDS yi, eri kum adihye, eri kum ndzifuo muma yɛ hwɛ ni yie oo wɔn hyɛ wo anku wo.

Let's be careful. AIDS is killing prominent people, royals, prophets. Let's be careful it doesn't come upon us and kill us. You are very important.

Daasebre Dwamena (Twi)

Yareɛ AIDS aa yɛhu scary adɔfo mesee hunhuhun. Married couples mu hwɛ muhu yie.
Daasebre mesu mɛ futuo nie.

AIDS is a scary disease, my dear ones.
Married couples, be careful.
Daasebre, this is my advice.

Chorus

All You can maintain one lover.
Shasha Marley Stick to a lover oh my people.
All It's not on it's not in.
Shasha Marley If it's not on, it's not in.
All You can wait until marriage.
Shasha Marley You can wait until marriage.
All Love life, Stop AIDS.
Shasha Marley Ooh ooh aah.
All You can maintain one lover.
Shasha Marley Ooh my brethren I say.
All It's not on it's not in.
Shasha Marley Watch where you going cause AIDS is real.
All You can wait until marriage.
Shasha Marley They've got no remedy.

All Love life.
Shasha Marley Got no remedy.
All Stop AIDS.
Shasha Marley What a killer disease.
All You can maintain one lover.
Shasha Marley Rastafari has come to warn you.
All It's not on it's not in.
Shasha Marley What a killer disease I say.
All You can wait until marriage.
Shasha Marley Stick to one lover what a killer disease I say.
All Love life, stop AIDS.
Shasha Marley Hear my cry oh mama.

Pete Pete (Vulture, Vulture) – A Traditional Fante Children's Song[1]

Fante	**English translation**
Pete, pete Senyiwa dedende senyiwa[2]	Vulture, vulture Senyiwa dedende senyiwa
Wo maame refre wo o Senyiwa dedende senyiwa	Your mother is calling you Senyiwa dedende senyiwa
Ose me me ye den? Senyiwa dedende senyiwa	What does she want me to do? Senyiwa dedende senyiwa
Ose be didi Senyiwa dedende senyiwa	She wants you to come and eat. Senyiwa dedende senyiwa
Ebere adziban a Senyiwa dedende senyiwa	What kind of food is it? Senyiwa dedende senyiwa
Fufu na abe nkwan Senyiwa dedende senyiwa	Fufu and palm nut soup Senyiwa dedende senyiwa
Mmofre ntse ndi o Senyiwa dedende senyiwa	Let the children share it. Senyiwa dedende senyiwa
Chorus (repeated several times)	
Senyiwa dedende Senyiwa dedende Senyiwa dedende senyiwa	Senyiwa dedende Senyiwa dedende Senyiwa dedende senyiwa

Annotations

[1] Visit YouTube (www.youtube.com/watch?app=desktop&v=oeUgsJkXPJQ) for a 1954 recording of Pete Pete, by Ivan Annan, for his album *Ghana: Children at Play: Children's Songs and Games*. Produced by Folkways Records. Song duration: 2.16 minutes].

[2] *Senyiwa dedende senyiwa* are nonsense words. Ghanaian ethnomusicologist J. H. Nketia (1958) notes that with these traditional Akan poems and songs "nonsense words are used mainly because of their rhythmic or prosodic interest" (p.10).

Song Title: Corona Virus

Artist: Kofi Kinaata
Source: (Official Video Published on 18 September 2020) https://youtu.be/hygo8Xrn4qc
Duration: 4 minutes, 19 seconds.
Languages: Fante, Ahanta, Ga, Ewe
Transcription: Henry Nii Adjiri Quarcoopome & Jemima Okai
Translation: English subtitles provided for the video

Video Intro Text

[Song is supported by Ministry of Fisheries and Aqua-culture Development, Commission of Fisheries, Ghana National Canoe Fishermen Council, National Fish Producers and Processors Association, University of Rhode Island, USAID]

***Voice-over introduction in English** – Excerpt from one of President Akufo Addo's COVID-19 addresses to the nation in his voice. "Fellow Ghanaians, the measures put in by government in response to the novel coronavirus disease, which has so affected, so far, one hundred and eighteen thousand people (118,000) on the globe. The WHO has now characterized it as a pandemic."*

Verse (Fante)

Coronavirus, COVID-19	Corona Virus, COVID-19
Mennfa ndi agorɔ koraa ooh, Wɔ yɛ huu	This virus is dangerous, don't joke with it.
Wo ayɛ merɛ, Fever na ɛbɔbɔ wo, w'abrɛ, wo ho na ɛdodɔ dodɔ wo	The symptoms are fever and coughing, tiredness, high temperature, loss of smell and tast; sore throat, loss of appetite.

Ɛbɛ hwɛ ɛnti scent, ɛnti taste, wo minemu ye wo yaa ooh, ɛntu mi ndzidzi.
Ɛbɛ rani na ɛnya cold, Ɛntumi ngye ahome oh, e feeli dizzy.
Ɔyɛ hu papaa
Yaliba ye wasiɛ bɛɛ bia
Asia wa kukumu nipa
Europe wa gugu ndwuma
Na Africa nso di agoro a, asem bɛ ba, hwɛ

You'll experience running stomach and cold, shortness of breath and feeling dizzy.
It's very scary!
This pandemic has destroyed a lot in the world.
In Asia it has killed multitudes
Even in Europe it has collapsed corporations.
So in Africa if we handle it with levity, it'll overwhelm us.

Refrain

Soldier suro corona
Lawyer ɔsuro corona
Malam suro corona
Wa la wo pastor yi ɔsuro corona.

The soldier is terrified of corona
The Lawyer is terrified of corona
The Mallam is terrified of corona
Even your own pastor is terrified of corona.

Chorus

Nia ye hu, nia y'ati, nti obia suro corona
Nia ye hu ooh, nia y'ati yen nyinaa yɛ suro corona
Nti wo nso suro corona

Because of what we've witnessed and heard, we are have terrified of corona.
Because of what we've witnessed and heard, we are have terrified of corona.
So you should also be terrified of Corona.

Verse (Fante)

Hyɛ wo nose mask sɛ ɛrekɔ kurom a
Men ma wo werɛ nfi wo two meters, Social distance wo ɛpo no na no
Hohro wo nsa fa samina yɛ
Hand sanitizer no fa bi fa yɛɛ
Men taa mpuwepuwe
Eni hwee yɛ a, n'atena fie
Seisei deɛ yen kyimakyima, by heart
Yɛn kyima mpo na yɛ hyia hyia, aha
Yɛn hyia mpo na yɛ kyia kyia
Nti gyae kasa tintin na twa ne tietia
Ko fie

Wear your nose mask when you're going out. Don't forget the two meter social distancing at the seashore.
Wash your hands with soap,
And don't forget to use hand sanitizers
If you don't have anything relevant to do out, stay home.
Irrelevant outing is now a thing of the past
So don't go out to exchange pleasantries
So keep the long conversations short and
go home

Chorus

Nia ye hu, nia y'ati, nti obia suro corona
Nia ye hu ooh, nia y'ati yen nyinaa yɛ suro corona
Nti wo nso suro corona

Because of what we've witnessed and heard, we are all terrified of corona.
Because of what we've witnessed and heard, we are all terrified of corona.

Verse (Nzema)

Sɛ ɛvo suonu na ɛkɔ wa do fɛlɛ
Kakyi ho kɛ coronavirus wɔkɛ
ɔdi kɛ ɛwura nose mask ni

So you should also be terrified of corona
Wear your nose mask when you're going out

Hwanhwan lele afa nguane ko di fɛlɛ
Pre mesia a moti yɛ w ɔfɛ
Fa social distance di dzinma wɔakɛ
Dabie tu corona nge nwodi lewula na moa pilee motwɛ

Don't forget the two meter social distancing at the seashore.
If you don't have anything relevant to do out, stay home

Verse (Ga)

Esumɔɔ ma nu akɛ, moko egbo shi wɔ ba nshɔ naa akɛ wɔyaa he loo.
Wolɛi akwɛ ni akɛ loo aka loo nokrokonkro.
Aunti Dedei wo onose mask.
Kɛ oshɛ nshɔ naa gbelemɔ distance.
Mɔni kɛɛ nshɔ nu akɛ tsaa Corona, kɛ okɛ ohiɛ fɔ henɔ noɛlɛɛ obaa gbo

I pray I don't hear of the death of any fisherfolk.
So the fisher folks should be mindful not to exchange the fish trading with something else.
Aunty Dedei, wear your nose mask and ensure social distancing always at the seashore.
Disregard the fallacy that the salty sea water cures Coronavirus.
So you should also be terrified of corona.

Verse (Ewe)

Evɔɖi loo, edɔbaɖae loo, amewuɖɔe loo, woyɔe na be Corona.
Kpele wo, kukugɛ la.
Eyata zã sanitizer, tɔdzi de la, akpa ƒlɛ la
Social distance loo. Elabe'ƒu yia me daa dɔɔ o.

Wear your nose mask when you're going out.
Don't forget to use hand sanitizers:
Don't forget the two meter social distancing at the seashore

Chorus (x1)

Verse (Fante)

Hwɛ asem kɛse frankaa nsidu
Nia wan ti apɔɔ hwɛ na afa na kɔ nsodu
Menfa wo vessels 'nsmuggle' nipa nmba Ghana
Nia aban aka mo ma yɛn hwɛ yi anidu
Herh yɛ sotie na hwɛ yie, didi yie
Di fruit na yɛ exercise na empo nsu no ɔnsa corona
Yɛn nom nsu no pii aa, na yɛn restie pii aa
Wo nfrɛ yee, yee mbrɛ
Ɛnya be a men pua, hyɛ dam hoa
Na frɛ numbers no na wo mbra bɛ fa wo
Me nsoro na ɛho no ntɛm deɛ ɔyɛ hu kora

Coming events cast their shadows.
Don't go fishing if you're feeling unwell.
Don't sneak people into Ghana with your vessel.
Let's adhere to the directives of the government. Be obedient and cautious; eat well. Take in a lot of fruit and exercise because the sea water doesn't cure corona. Let's drink a lot of water and rest well.
Regards to the fisherfolks.
If you experience the symptoms stay indoors and call the numbers for prompt response because when it's diagnosed early it's not as dangerous.

Chorus (x1)
Refrain (x1)
Chorus (x1)

Song Title: Corona

Artist: Tulenkey
Source: Tulenkey on Youtube (Published on 24 March 2020) www.youtube.com/watch?v=FFFy8UNleoU
Duration: 3 minutes, 42 seconds
Languages: Twi, Pidgin English
Transcription and annotations: Jemima Okai
Translation: Ama de-Graft Aikins

Twi/Pidgin English	English translation
Ya cancel obia shows, ya close close dwom	All the shows are cancelled, all the clubs are closed
Tule[1] paa anka weekend bia me booku last flight kɔ Oseikrom[2]	Tule, who, every weekend would have booked the last flight to Oseikrom
Nso ya cancel shows, I for stay home	But the shows are cancelled, I have to stay home
Me cash kraa locki, I make merɛ	My cash is locked, I am weak
kɔ hwɛ Mole[3] ne MP[3] they make slow	See Mole and MP, they are now slow
Fameye[3] nso dodge promoters	Fameye is dodging promoters
Corona nti wo bɔ'wa na obia suro	Because of corona, if you cough everyone is afraid
Corona nti wo hyia me na y'a ma me blow	Because of corona, when you meet me give a fist bump
Corona nti Ronaldo atu akɔ hyɛ Island	Because of corona Ronaldo is hiding on an island
Whan na ensuro, obia suro'wuo	Who isn't afraid, everyone is afraid of death
Liverpool shiishii, them make merɛ	Even brash Liverpool, is now weak
Oswald and friends all make merɛ	Oswald and friends are all weak
And the boys wey	And the boys who
take thema fees buy stand for Repu[4]	Use their fees to buy a stand at Repu
only God can save them	Only God can save them
I can't go out	
I can't go out	
I'm so alone now	
I miss Bloom bar	
I miss Bloom bar	
I want to chill now	
Want to bɔɔling[5] oooooo	
I want to link up	

I want to turn up! Turn up! Turn up!	
Cure! Where is the cure baby	
Life start dey bore lately	
What is on the news	
Everyday all day bad news sɔnn[6]	
Wash your hands whilst there is no cure baby	Wash your hands whilst there is no cure baby
Sanitize be strong baby	Sanitize be strong baby
Nyame te asi yi deɛ	As long as God lives
Our nation no go fall	Our nation will not fall
Corona I hate what you doing!	Corona I hate what you doing!
Wo ne China wɔ beef aa ɛnfa'mba yɛn so ooo	If you have beef with China, don't involve us
We are peaceful people	We are peaceful people
Corona stop what you doing	Corona stop what you doing
Shame on you mmerewa foɔ na wo pɛ,	Shame on you targeting elderly women
they are feeble people	they are feeble people
Corona, hate what you doing	
Stop what you doing	
Corona	
Corona	
Corona, hate what you doing	
Stop what you doing	
Corona	
Corona	
Yɛte hɔ aa mo se bird flu (bird flu)	At first you all said Bird Flu (bird flu)
Ankyɛ na mose swine flu (swine flu)	Soon after you said Swine Flu (swine flu)
Yɛbɛ te yɛ anni aaa rabies (rabies)	Before we realised it was rabies (rabies)
Yɛda ne yɛn ho aa HIV (mokoraa adɛn?)	We turned around, HIV (what is it with you all!)
Afei na corona (rona)	Right now it is corona (rona)
Saa na mo yɛɛ ebolo (bola)	Same way you made Ebola (bola)
White man always tryna find ways to eradicate black population	
Oh no	
Leave the black alone	
Why do you kill your own?	
Global war but everybody jie eye[7] dey protect their own	
We should come together	
That's when we stand a chance so my friend	
This no bi the time to point fingers	
The thing dey spread	

(Corona) try not to touch your face
(Corona) sanitize your hands
(Corona) try and keep your distance
  when you are talking to a friend
(Corona), always wash your hands
(Corona) try and stay indoors
(Corona) neɛ duru yi deɛ yɛ'nidasoɔ
  nyinaa towards the Lord
(Corona) I hate what you doing
Wo ne China wɔ beef aa ɛnfa ɛmba yɛn
  so ooo
We are peaceful people
Corona stop what you doing
Shame on you mmerewa foɔ na wo pɛ,
they are feeble people
Corona, hate what you doing
Stop what you doing
Corona
Corona
Corona, hate what you doing
Stop what you doing
Corona
Corona
Heal the world make it a better place,
make it a better place (2x)

Annotations

[1] Tule – Tulenkey.
[2] Oseikrom – translation Osei's Town – is a local name for Kumasi. Osei refers to Osei Tutu I, one of the founders of the Asante Empire and the first King of Asante (Asantehene), ruling between 1695 and 1717.
[3] Mole, MP and Fameye are hiplife artists.
[4] 'Repu' is short for Republic. Here Tulenkey was referring to the popular hall week of Republic Hall, KNUST.
[5] Balling: Hip Hop derived slang for partying or chilling.
[6] Sɔnn – too much, a lot, in Ga.
[7] Jie eye – ignore, pretend not to see.

APPENDIX 3C.

Agbeve Herbal Clinic Advert

An Agbeve Clinic mobile van advert, recorded on Friday, 14 July, 2023, 6 am, in Osu, Accra.

Recording by: Dennis Obuobi
Duration: 2 minutes, 43 seconds
Language: Ga
Transcription and translation: Ruth Anokye

Ga	
Ebaaha ni ohe ajɔbo fiofio obaana akɛ ohela nɛɛ eje jɛmɛ kraa. Tsofa ni wɔ jieɔ eyi ji, Agbeve tonic ehi kɛ ha mɔ fɛɛ mɔ	You'll feel relieved. You'll gradually come to understand that your condition will eventually go away. Agbeve tonic is the medication we are recommending to you; it is beneficial for everyone.
Gbekɛbii ni yɛ kwashiorkor obaaná ni emusuŋ ebama ehie gɛdɛmoo, nakai gbekɛ kɛ enaagbai nɛ wɔ baahã lɛ Agbeve sweet tonic kɛ eko ni enu	We shall provide Agbeve sweet tonic to a child who has Kwashiorkor (micro-nutrient deficiency condition) to drink.
Gbekɛbii ekomɛi ayee niyenii akpa, amɛ yiteŋ fɛɛ feɔ framframfram, kɛ onaagbã ji enɛ, tsi obɛŋkɛ wɔ, wɔ baa ha bo agbeve tonic kɛ eko ko ni onu	Some children eat an imbalanced meal diet and have thin, weak hair on their heads. If you visit us with this problem, we are going to give you Agbeve tonic to drink.
Yeimeji ni amɛɛ ye tswi tsetse, yeimei ni anyɛɛ shi ate jogbaŋŋ, kɛ gbɔmɔ te shi ja emɔmɔ gbogboi amli ni etawɔ tso ni ekɛ nyiɛ. Nakutsei ɛ fɛɛ mli egbɔjɔ loo, enu he akɛ ewa ehe aloo, mɛi ni amɛtsui tswaa fe nine loo, mɛi ni amɛlá nɔ kɔɔ fe nine. Nɛkɛ helai nɛɛ fɛɛ ba, wɔ ba ha bo agbeve tonic kɛ eko, ebaa saa bo, ebaa ha ni ofee fɛɛfɛo. Agbeve tonic, yareɛ bɛkɔ.	Older women with rheumatism, those with knee problems or weak knees who require aid to stand or walk, and those with an elevated heartbeat or high blood pressure should visit us for Agbeve tonic; it will heal them and make them attractive.
	Agbeve tonic, cure for illness

Mɛi komɛi hu amɛhiŋmɛii, ni ji hiŋmɛii nɔ feɔ kusuu. . .enaa nii jogbaŋŋ, enyɛɛ wolo ekane. Biblia ni akaneɔ nɛɛ enyɛɛ eko ekane. Kɛ onaagbã nɛɛ, tsi obɛŋkɛ wɔ ni wɔ ha bo tsofa. Obaana hejɔlɛ loo, wɔ helatsamɔhe ni yɔɔ Suotuom.

Wɔ yɛ tsɔnei ni akɛ kwɛɔ gbɔmɔtso hei fɛɛ ni hela eyatee tee amɛhe yɛɛ, wɔ baa na ni wɔ baa ha bo tsofa. Tsi obɛŋkɛ wɔ ko ni wɔ ha bo agbeve tonic kɛ eko. No ɛɛ blema tsofa ni, ni etsaa helai fɛɛ helai, tsi obɛŋkɛ wɔ.

Helai komei hu ni ehenɔ sikli hela nɛkɛ. Sikli helai sɛɛkpenɛɛ he mɔmɔɔ kɛ gbekɛbii fɛɛ, nɔ ni wɔtsɛɔ akɛ diabetes. kɛ ji akɛ onaagbã nɛɛ, tsi obɛŋkɛ wɔ, wɔ baa ha bo agbeve tonic.

Diabetes nɛɛ kɛ emɔ bo bei babaoo. Akɛɛ okadii ekomei ni akɛ naa ekolɛ ni najii ɛ fuɔ, kɛ otsu nii fio oonu he akɛ etɔ bo. Eje akɛ kɛ onyiɛ kɛ jɛ biɛ kɛ shɛ biɛ nɔɔ otsui baa tswa waa diɛŋtsɛ . Kɛ onaagbã nɛɛ, tsi obɛŋkɛ wɔ, tsi obɛŋkɛ wɔ, wɔ baa ha bo agbeve tonic kɛ eko.

Tsofa nɛɛ kɛ onu ɛ, kɛ ebote ogbɔmɔtso mli, ebaa fɔ ola mli ni ebaa ha ni kɔɔyɔɔ atsu nii jogbaŋŋ ni hei fɛɛ ni sane la ashɛ yɛ ogbɔmɔtso mli, ebaa tsu nii pɛpɛɛpɛ. Bei fio sɛɛ, obaa na akɛ ohe efee fɛɛfɛɔ

Kɛ yoofoyo ji bo, otee fɔmɔ oba ni ooha bi fufɔ baa ni na wɔ, kɛ wɔ agba sane, wɔ baa ha bo gbɛtsɔɔmɔ ni kɔɔ tsofa nɛɛ kɛ he numɔ he

Tsofã ehi ha mɔfɛɛmɔ ni ehi ha helai fɛɛ helai ni yieɔ bo ɛ, tsi obɛŋkɛ wɔ, wɔ baa ha bo agbeve tonic kɛ eko.

Oyitso ni gbaa ona?

– fading audio –

Some people struggle to read books or the Bible because of foggy eyesight, poor vision, or both. If this is a problem for you, please see us and we'll offer you some medicine to help, or come to our hospital in Soutuom.

We can diagnose your complete body and treat you with cutting-edge, effective technologies.

Come to us, and we will give you Agbeve tonic, an ancient remedy that treats all ailments and diseases. Visit us.

You can come to us and receive Agbeve tonic if you have diabetes. Diabetes is one illness that presently affects both young and old people.

Swollen legs, exhaustion, and an accelerated heartbeat are a few of the signs and symptoms of diabetes. Visit us for Agbeve tonic.

When you take this medication, it will enter your bloodstream, cleanse it, and help your veins and arteries work properly so that blood can flow to all of your body's vital organs without interruption. You will quickly develop a stunning appearance.

Come to us if you are a lactating mother, and we will advise you on how to use and take this medication.

It is good for everybody and cures all illnesses. We will provide you with the Agbeve tonic if you come to us.

Do you frequently experience headaches?

APPENDIX 3D.

'Corona ABCD' Comedy Sketch

Comedian: Clemento Suarez
Source: Published on Instagram on 3 April 2020 – www.instagram.com/tv/B-iGjAonSCu/?igshid=MDJmNzVkMjY=
Duration: 3 minutes, 16 seconds
Languages: Twi, Twinglish, Fantenglish, English
Transcription: Francis Agyei
Translation and annotations: Francis Agyei and Ama de-Graft Aikins

Journalist: Herh School Boy eee, Timothy bra bra . . . eei ... Timothy ɛtesɛn?	Journalist: Hey, school boy, Timothy, come, come here. . ..ei Timothy how are you?
Timothy: Mepawokyɛw ɛyɛ oo	Timothy: Please fine ooo
Journalist: eee ahaa Timothy ka corona ABCD no kyerɛ me	Journalist: eee ahaa Timothy, tell me the corona ABCDTimothy:
Timothy: Hehe . . . Colonial ABCD[1]	Hehe. . .Colonial ABCD
A: Abroso ooo, abɔ yɛ so! ama afei yɛ hyehyɛ dan mu	A: It's gone overboard ooo. We don't know what to do with it. Now, we are only in our rooms
B: Bibiara ɛnnyɛ me ehi sɛ, yɛ bɔ wa dada nɛnso sɛ ɛnɛ, ntɛsuo twi wo koraa a, nna obi pɛ wo abɔ wo dua.	B: Nothing annoys me more than the fact that we have always had our coughs. But today, even if saliva chokes you, then somebody wants to curse you.
C: Colona vilus, Nyame betua wo ka.	C: Colona vilus, God will punish you
D: Didi yie ooo menua Kwame, didi yie na fa vitamin A, B, C, D, E, F . . .	D: Eat well ooo my brother Kwame. Eat well and take vitamins A, B, C, D, E, F..
E: Eii, nti Prince Charles aa ɛndra yiara onyaa bi no, ne ho atɔ no. ɛnieɛ, me nua Allotey hyɛ fie ooo na wonni hwee	E: Eii so Prince Charles who contracted the disease only yesterday has recovered? Then Allotey my brother, you need to stay home, because you don't have anything.

F: Fri me so kɔ koraa ana wo anbɛma me yareɛ no bi	F: Get away from me, before you infect me with the disease
G: Gyae gyimie no na tena fie	G: Stop fooling around and stay home
H: Hohoro wonsa, fa samina yɛ, hohoro wonsa, fa samina ka, hohoro wonsa ooo hohoro wonsa ooo fa samena yɛ, saa na ɛyɛ[2]	H: Wash your hand, use soap , wash your hands, use soap, wash your hands ooo, wash your hands ooo, use soap.. That is right
I: I don't fear huu, colona no . . .	I: I don't fear anything, that colona
J: June deɛ na obia ɛwu	J: By June, everybody would have died
Journalist: Hey, fa wo ano ka nsɛm pa	Journalist: Hey, use your mouth to say good things
Timothy: J – JJ time na yɛse tena fie anka woaa nka wo bɛte[3]	Timothy: J – if it were during JJ's time that you were told to stay at home, you would see
K: Kai oo sɛ efutusɛm se, wo sɔre anopa aa nom nsuo na tena fie!	K: Remember that, the advice is , when you wake up in the morning, drink water and stay at home
L: Lockdown aa wose 'na me dwene sɛ president se yenkɔ tɔn credit' na wo tɔn ama hwan?[4]	L: (We are on) Lockdown, then you say 'I thought the president said we can go and sell credit'. Who are you selling to?
M: Mmmm adiɛ no ani ayɛ nyan	M: Mmmm the thing has gotten really serious
N: Nokware nokware mese mo sɛ obiaa nnyɛ ma danfo nti wohu me aa twam!	N: Verily verily, I say unto you, nobody is my friend so when you see me just pass
O: Ooo by June deɛ na	O: Ohhh by June then. . .. . .
Journalist: Hey hey hey . . . sesa mu!	Journalist: Hey hey hey. . ..change that!
Timothy: O – Opambuor, Owusu-Bempah, Oduro, Obɔfuɔ ne Obinim, bebiara a ɔmo wɔ dier, obi nnim [5]	Timothy: O – Opambour, Owusu-Bempah, Oduro, Ɔbɔfoɔ [*referring to Rev. Obofour*] and Obinim, whatever they have nobody knows.
P: Petre petre saa na woanya yareɛ no bi	P: Keep rushing and rushing,you will contract the disease
Q: Quarantine, nyɛ ne nua ne Valentine nti no ma girl no nkɔ fie	Q: Quarantine is not a sibling to Valentine, so let the girl go home
R: Rest in peace, ɔmo a ɔmo awu no nyinaa. Wo wɔ fie nsoso aa, rest in peace!	R: Rest in peace, all those who are dead. If you are at home, you too rest in peace!
S: Still by June deɛ na obiara awu . . .	S: Still by June then everybody. . .. . .
Journalist: Oh change no	Journalist: Oh change it
Timothy: By June dier . . .	Timothy: By June. . ..
Journalist: Change no!	Journalist: Change it

Timothy: S – Science student aa woagyimi sei koraa deɛ me nnhuu bi da! Hyɛ dan mu aa wose, 'I am a science student'. Wo lecturer koraa ada, na wo a wo kɔ twerɛ IA

Timothy: S – I've never seen such a foolish science student before. They say stay inside, you say "I am a science student". Even your lecturer is asleep, how much more you who are going write an IA

T: Tete wɔ bi ka aa, tete wɔ bi kyerɛ. Yɛn maame ne yɛn Papa no de 83 kɔm no na atwa yɛn ntrɔ saa sɛ yɛnso yenya bi[6]

T: If history has something to say, history has something to teach. Our mothers and fathers have used the 1983 famine to bamboozle us for so long. Now we have also got our famine.

U: U and I were not there papa yi dier, asem yi siiyɛ no deɛ menntee ne nka kolaa

U: The U and I were not there man , as for him, when this thing happened, I haven't heard from him at all

V: Veli veli, I say unto you, tena fie!

V: Verily verily I say unto you, stay at home

W: Woa wo bɔ wa ne woa wo wensew, kata wo ano, kata wo hwene

W: Those of you who cough and those who sneeze, close your mouth, cover your nose

X: X-ray kraa ntumi nhu aboa no ooo, Yoo

X: Even X-ray cannot see the virus ooo, Yoo

Journalist: Y?

Journalist: 'Y'?

Timothy: Sɛ maka 'Yoo' deda[7]

Timothy: But I have said 'Yoo' already

Z: Zongo minister no ɔwɔ hɔ? Mmm[8]

Z: The Zongo minister, is s/he there? Mmm

Journalist: Ei wo ayɛ adeɛ, wo ayɛ adeɛ. Bɔ wo nsa mu ma wo ho.

Journalist: Ei. . .you have done well, you have done well. Clap for yourself

Timothy: Ahaa, ma me sika . . .

Timothy: Ahaa. . .give me money

Annotations

[1] Colonial ABCD – extension of Twinglish version of 'corona virus'. Other Twinglish examples – colona, veli veli.

[2] Hohorowonsa song – from the Truly Clean Hands Campaign (see Scott et al. 2008; Chapter 3). The song lyrics also appear in Kofi Kinaata's COVID-19 song.

[3] JJ – former president of Ghana, Flight Lieutenant Jerry John Rawlings.

[4] The credit sellers – phone credit.

[5] Opambuor, Owusu-Bempah, Oduro, Obɔfuɔ ne Obinim – all prominent Pentecostal Charismatic Church leaders. In the early

months of the pandemic, their messaging to their congregants was that Christian faith would protect them from contracting COVID-19. They also lobbied, unsuccessfully, against the government's decision to impose lockdown as that would affect church attendance. The implicit meaning of 'whatever they have' is whatever they have that protects them from COVID-19 infection.

[6] '83' – refers to the 1983 famine.

[7] Yoo – OK.

[8] The Zongo Minister – a new and controversial ministerial portfolio established by the NPP government that aimed to address poverty in urban migrant communities.

References

Abdulla, Sharifa (2016). The use of folk media: a contradictory discourse. *Research in Drama Education: The Journal of Applied Theatre and Performance*, 21(4), 459–464.

Acquah, Emmanuel O. (2016). Choral singing and wellbeing: Findings from a survey of the mixed-chorus experience from music students of the University of Education Winneba, Ghana. *Legon Journal of the Humanities*, 27(2), 1–3.

Adams, Glenn and Dzokoto, Vivian (2003). Self and identity in African studies. *Self and Identity*, 2(4), 345–359.

Addo-Fening, Robert (2013). Ghana under colonial rule: An outline of the early period and the interwar years. *Transactions of the Historical Society of Ghana*, 15, 39–70.

Adjei, Sela K. (2020). Abstraction and the sublime in art: Bridging the gap between 'modern art' and Ewe Vodu aesthetics. *The Garage Journal: Studies in Art, Museums & Culture*, 01, 162–187.

Adjonyoh, Zoe (2017). *Zoe's Ghana Kitchen: Traditional Recipes Remixed for the Modern Kitchen*. London: Octopus Publishing Group Ltd.

Agyei-Mensah, Samuel (2001). Twelve years of HIV/AIDS in Ghana: Puzzles of interpretation. *Canadian Journal of African Studies*, 35(3), 441–472.

Akyeampong, Emmanuel (1995). Alcoholism in Ghana: A sociocultural exploration. *Culture, Medicine and Psychiatry*, 19(2), 261–280.

(2002). Bukom and the social history of boxing in Accra: Warfare and citizenship in Precolonial Ga Society. *The International Journal of African Historical Studies*, 5(1), 39–60.

Alidu, Seidu, Dankyi, Ernestina and Tsiboe-Darko, Antoinette (2016). Aging policies in Ghana: A review of the Livelihood Empowerment against Poverty and the National Health Insurance Scheme. *Ghana Studies*, 19(1), 154–172.

Allman, Jean (1994). Making mothers: Missionaries, medical officers and women's work in colonial Asante, 1924–1945. *History Workshop*, 38(1), 23–47.

Alviso, Ric (2011). Tears run dry: Coping with AIDS through music in Zimbabwe. In G. Barz and J. M. Cohen (eds.), *The Culture of AIDS in Africa: Hope and Healing through Music and the Arts*. Oxford: Oxford University Press (pp. 56–62).

Amoah, Patrick, Drechsel, Pay, Abaidoo, Robert C. and Ntow, William J. (2006). Pesticide and pathogen contamination of vegetables in Ghana's urban markets. *Archives of Environmental Contamination and Toxicology*, 50, 1–6.

Ampomah, Kingsley (2014). An investigation into Adowa and Adzewa music and dance of the Akan People of Ghana. *International Journal of Humanities and Social Science*, 4(10), 117–124.

Ansu-Kyeremeh, Kwasi, Richter, Magdalena, Vallianatos, Helen, et al. (2016). Rural women's exposure to health messages and understandings of health. *Journal of Health Communication*, 1(3).

Appiah, Kwame Anthony (1992). *In My Father's House: Africa in the Philosophy of Culture*. Oxford: Oxford University Press.

Appiah, Peggy, Appiah, Kwame Anthony and Agyemang-Duah, Ivor (2008). *Bu me Bɛ: Proverbs of the Akans*. Banbury: Ayebia Clarke Publishing.

Assefa, Yibeltal, Gilks, Charles F., van de Pas, Remco, et al. (2021). Reimagining global health systems for the 21st century: Lessons from the COVID-19 pandemic. *BMJ Global Health*, 6(4), e004882.

Atobrah, Deborah (2016). Elderly women, community participation, and family care in Ghana: Lessons from HIV response and AIDS Orphan Care in Manya Krobo. *Ghana Studies*, 19(1), 73–94.

Awenva, A. D., Read, Ursula M., Ofori-Atta, Angela L., et al. (2010). From mental health policy development in Ghana to implementation: What are the barriers? *African Journal of Psychiatry*, 13(3), 184–191.

Awusabo-Asare, Kofi, Abane, Albert M., Badasu, D., et al. (1999). 'All die be die': obstacles to change in the face of HIV infection in Ghana. In John Charles Caldwell (ed.), *Resistances to Behavioural Change to Reduce HIV/AIDS Infection in Predominantly Heterosexual Epidemics in Third World Countries*. Canberra: Health Transition Centre/Australian National University (pp. 125–132).

Ayettey, A. S., Quakyi, Isabella, A., Ayettey-Annie, H. N. G., et al. (2020). Rapid response: A case for hydrogen peroxide mouthwash and gargle to limit SARS-CoV-2 infection. *BMJ*, 368, m1252rr-27.

Ba, Amadou Hampate (1976). African art: Where the hand has ears. In The UNESCO Courier, XXIX, 2 (537), pp. 12–19.

Bannister, David (2021). The Sorcerer's Apprentice: Sleeping sickness, onchocerciasis, and unintended consequences in Ghana, 1930–60. *The Journal of African History*, 62(1), 29–57.

Barber, Karin (1987). Popular arts in Africa. *African Studies Review*, 30(3), 1–78.

Barnor, Mathew A. (2001). *A Socio-Medical Adventure in Ghana: Autobiography of Dr. M. A. Barnor*. Mampong-Akuapem, Ghana: Viesco Universal.

Barz, Gregory and Cohen, Judah M. (2011). *The Culture of AIDS in Africa: Hope and Healing through Music and the Arts*. Oxford: Oxford University Press.

Basher, T., Elhakim, A. S., el Fawal, K., et al. (1983). On vagrancy and psychosis. *Community Mental Health Journal*, 19(1), 27–41.

Beck, Rose Marie (2006). Popular media for HIV/AIDS prevention? Comparing two comics: Kingo and the Sara Communication Initiative. *The Journal of Modern African Studies*, 44(4), 513–541.

Ben-Amos, Paula (1989). African visual arts from a social perspective. *African Studies Review*, 32(2), 1–53.

Blier, Suzanne Preston (1993). Truth and seeing: Magic, custom and fetish in art history. In Robert H. Bates, V. Y. Mudimbe and Jean O'Barr (eds.), *Africa and the Disciplines: The Contributions of Research in Africa to the Social Sciences and Humanities*. Chicago: University of Chicago Press (pp. 139–166).

Boal, Augusto (1992). *Games for Actors and Non-Actors*. London: Routledge.

Bob-Milliar, George M. (2009). Chieftaincy, diaspora and development: The institution of Nkosuohene in Ghana. *African Affairs*, 108(433), 541–558.

Boneh, Gail and Jaganath, Devan (2011). Performance as a component of HIV/AIDS education: Process and collaboration for empowerment and discussion. *American Journal of Public Health*, 101(3), 455–464.

Booker, Nancy Achieng, Miller, Ann Neville and Ngure, Peter (2016). Heavy sexual content versus safer sex content: A content analysis of the entertainment education drama Shuga. *Health Communication*, 31, 1437–1446.

Bosompra, Kwadwo (2007–2008). The potential of drama and songs as channels for AIDS education in Africa: A report on focus group findings from Ghana. *International Quarterly of Community Health Education*, 28(2), 127–151.

Bosu, William (2012). A comprehensive review of the policy and programmatic response to chronic non-communicable disease in Ghana. *Ghana Medical Journal*, 46(2), 69–78.

Boulay, Mark, Tweedie, Ian and Fiagbey, Emmanuel (2008). The effectiveness of a national communication campaign using religious leaders to reduce HIV-related stigma in Ghana. *African Journal of AIDS Research*, 7(1), 133–141.

Breidenbach, Paul S. (1976). Colour symbolism and ideology in a Ghanaian Healing Movement. *Africa*, 46(2), 137–145.

Bunn, Christopher, Kalinga, Chisomo, Mtema, Otiyela, et al. (2020). Arts-based approaches to promoting health in sub-Saharan Africa: A scoping review. *BMJ Global Health*, 5(5), e001987.

Campbell, Catherine (2003). *Letting Them Die: Why HIV/AIDS Prevention Programmes Fail*. Oxford: James Currey.

Campbell, Catherine and Scott, Kerry (2011). Mediated health campaigns: From information to social change. In Hook Derek, Franks Bradley and Bauer Martin (eds.), *Social Psychology of Communication*. Basingstoke: Palgrave. (pp. 266–283).

Campbell, C., Nair, Y. and Maimane, S. (2007). Building contexts that support effective community responses to HIV/AIDS: A South African case study. *American Journal of Community Psychology*, 39(3–4), 347–363.

Carl, Florian and Kutsidzo, Rosemond (2016). Music and wellbeing in everyday life: An exploratory study of music experience in Ghana. *Legon Journal of the Humanities*, 27(2), 29–46.

Cataliotti, Robert (2022). *Drumsville!: The Evolution of the New Orleans Beat*. Baton Rouge: LSU Press.

Chambers, Robert (1997). *Whose Reality Counts? Putting the Last First*. London: IT Publications.

Charmaz, Cathy (1983). Loss of self: A fundamental form of suffering in the chronically ill. *Sociology of Health and Illness*, 15(2), 168–195.

Chinyowa, Kennedy C. (2015). Participation as 'repressive myth': A case study of the Interactive Themba Theatre Organisation in South Africa. *Research in Drama Education: The Journal of Applied Theatre and Performance*, 20(1), 12–23.

Chu, Valerie (2010). Within the box: Cross-cultural art therapy with survivors of the Rwanda Genocide. *Art Therapy: Journal of the American Art Therapy Association*, 27(1), 4–10.

Clark, Gracia (1994). *Onions Are My Husband: Survival and Accumulation By West African Market Women*. Chicago: University of Chicago Press.

Cole, Herbet M. and Ross, Doran H. (1977). *The Arts of Ghana*. Berkeley, CA: University of California Press.

Collins, John (1976). Comic Opera in Ghana. *African Arts*, 9(2), 50–57.

(2017). Popular performance and culture in Ghana: The past 50 years. *Ghana Studies*, 20(1), 175–219.

Cornish, Flora, Breton, Nancy, Moreno-Tabarez, U., et al. (2023). Participatory action research. *Nature Research Methods Primer*, 3(34), 1–14.

Costa, Lucy, Voronka, Jijian, Landry, Danielle, et al. (2012). 'Recovering our stories': A small act of resistance. *Studies in Social Justice*, 6(1), 85–101.

Crossley, Michele L. (2000). *Rethinking Health Psychology*. Buckingham: Open University Press.

Dakubu, Mary Esther Kropp (1990). Why spider is king of stories: The message in the medium of a West African tale. *African Languages and Cultures*, 3(1), 33–56.

Davies, Thom (2022). Slow violence and toxic geographies: 'Out of sight' to whom? *Environment and Planning C: Politics and Space*, 40(2), 409–427.

de-Graft Aikins, Ama (2005). Social Representations of Diabetes in Ghana: Reconstructing Self, Society and Culture. Unpublished PhD Thesis, London School of Economics and Political Science.

(2006). Reframing applied disease stigma research: A multilevel analysis of diabetes stigma in Ghana. *Journal of Community and Applied Social Psychology*, 16(6), 426–441.

(2009). Out of your mind? Exploring the role of creative arts in mental health promotion and rehabilitation in Ghana. *New Legon Observer*, 3(2), 8–12.

(2010). Beyond "food is medicine": Evaluating the impact of Ghana's Regenerative Health and Nutrition Pilot Programme. *Ghana Social Science Journal*, 7(1), 14–35.

(2011). Culture, diet and the maternal body: Ghanaian women's perspectives on food, fat and childbearing. In Maya Unnithan-Kumar and Soraya Tremayne (eds.), *Fatness and the Maternal Body: Women's Experiences of Corporeality and the Shaping of Social Policy*. Oxford: Berghahn Books (pp. 130–154).

(2012). Familiarising the unfamiliar: Cognitive polyphasia, emotions and the creation of social representations. *Papers on Social Representations*, 21, 7.1–7.28.

(2015). Mental illness and destitution in Ghana: a social psychological perspective. In Emmanuel Akyeampong, Alan Hill and Arthur Kleinman (eds.), *The Culture of Mental Illness and Psychiatric Practice in Africa*. Bloomington: Indiana University Press (pp. 112–143).

(2020). "Colonial virus"? Creative arts and public understanding of COVID-19 in Ghana. *Journal of the British Academy*, 8, 401–413.

de-Graft Aikins, Ama, Boynton, Petra and Atanga, Lilian L. (2010). Developing effective chronic disease prevention in Africa: Insights from Ghana and Cameroon. *Globalization and Health*, 6, 6.

de-Graft Aikins, Ama and Koram, Kwadwo (2017). Health and healthcare in Ghana, 1957–2017. In E. Aryeetey and R. Kanbur (eds.), *The Economy of Ghana: Sixty Years after Independence*. Oxford: Oxford University Press (pp. 365–384).

de Graft Aikins, Ama and Akoi-Jackson, Bernard (2020). "Colonial virus": COVID-19, creative arts and public health communication in Ghana. *Ghana Medical Journal*, 54(3), 86–96.

de-Graft Aikins, Ama, Kushitor, Mawuli, Boatemaa, Sandra, et al. (2020). Building cardiovascular disease (CVD) competence in an urban poor Ghanaian community: A social psychology of participation approach. *Journal of Community and Applied Social Psychology*, 30(4), 419–440.

de-Graft Aikins, Ama, Sanuade, Olutobi, Agyei, Francis, Bewong, R. Fatric and Akoi-Jackson, Bernard (2024). Applying arts to health interventions and health research in Ghana: A scoping review. *Arts & Health*, 1–20.

de-Graft Aikins, Ama, Sanuade, Olutobi, Baatiema, et al. (2021). COVID-19, chronic conditions and structural poverty: A social psychological assessment of the needs of a vulnerable community in Accra, Ghana. *Journal of Social and Political Psychology*, 9(2), 577–591.

de-Graft Aikins, Ama, Sanuade, Olutobi, Baatiema, Leonard, et al. (2023). How chronic conditions are understood, experienced and managed within African communities in Europe, North America and Australia: A synthesis of qualitative studies. *PLoS One*, 18(2), e0277325.

de Witte, Marleen (2011). Of corpses, clay, and photographs: Body imagery and changing technologies of remembrance in Asante funeral culture. In Michael Jindra and Joël Noret (eds.), *Funerals in Africa: Explorations of a Social Phenomenon*. Oxford: Berghahn Books (pp. 177–206).

Downes, Catherine, Philip, Keir E. J., Lewis, Adam, et al. (2019). Singing for breathing Uganda: Group singing for people with chronic lung disease in Kampala. *Journal of Applied Arts & Health*, 10(2), 219–228.

Droney, Damien (2022). Alternative medicine devices and the making of scientific herbal medicine in Ghana. *Postcolonial Studies*, 25(2), 229–247.

Du Bois, W. E. B. ([1903] 1965). *The Souls of Black Folk*. London: Longmans, Green & Co.

Duodu, Cameron (2004). The fear of vaccines. *New African*, 428, 50–55.

Eribo, Shaninomi (2021). COVID-19 and African Civil Society Organizations: impact and responses. in *Alliance for African Partnership Perspectives, Volume*

1: African Universities and the COVID-19 Pandemic (Special Issue). East Lansing, MI: Alliance for African Partnership - Michigan State University (pp. 147–155).

Evans, Freddi Williams (2011). *Congo Square: African Roots in New Orleans.* Lafayette: University of Louisiana at Lafayette Press.

Fancourt, Daisy and Finn, S. (2019). *What Is the Evidence on the Role of the Arts in Improving Health and Well-Being? A Scoping Review.* Switzerland: WHO.

Fanon, Franz (1963). *The Wretched of the Earth.* New York: Grove Press.

Faria, Caroline (2008). Privileging prevention, gendering responsibility: An analysis of the Ghanaian campaign against HIV/AIDS. *Social & Cultural Geography*, 9(1), 41–73.

Feldman-Savelsberg, Pamela, Ndonko, Flavien T. and Schmidt-Ehry, Bergis (2000). Sterilizing vaccines or the politics of the Womb: Retrospective study of a rumor in Cameroon. *Medical Anthropology Quarterly*, 14(2), 159–179.

Fernandez Olmos, Margarite and Paravisini-Gebert, Lizabeth (2022). *Creole Religions of the Caribbean: From Vodou and Santeria to Obeah and Espiritismo.* New York: New York University Press.

Field, M. J. (1937). *Religion and Medicine of the Ga People.* Oxford: Oxford University Press.

Fortes, Meyer (1981). Tallensi children's drawings. In B. Lloyd and J. Gay (eds.), *Universals of Human Thought: Some African Evidence.* Cambridge: Cambridge University Press (pp. 46–70).

Foss, Katherine A. (2020). How the 1918 Pandemic Got Meme-ified in Jokes, Songs and Poems. www.smithsonian.mag.com/history/memes-1918-pandemic (last accessed 26th September 2023).

Foucault, Michel (1988). Technologies of the self. In L. Martin, H. Gutman and P. Hutton (eds.), *Technologies of the Self: A Seminar with Michel Foucault.* Amherst: University of Massachusetts Press (pp. 16–49).

Frank, Lauren B., Murphy, Sheila T., Chatterjee, Joyee S., et al. (2015). Telling stories, saving lives: Creating narrative health messages. *Health Communication*, 30(2): 154–163.

Freire, Paulo (1970/2017). *Pedagogy of the Oppressed.* New York: Penguin RandomHouse.

Frishkopf, Michael, Hamze, Hasan, Alhassan, Mubarak, et al. (2016). Performing arts as a social technology for community health promotion in northern Ghana. *Family Medicine and Community Health*, 4(1), 22–36.

Frishkopf, Michael, Zakus, David, Hamze, Hasan, et al. (2016). Traditional music as a sustainable social technology for Community Health Promotion in Africa: "Singing and Dancing for Health" in rural Northern Ghana. *Legon Journal of the Humanities*, 27(2), 47–72.

Galtung, Johan (1969). Violence, peace, and peace research. *Journal of Peace Research*, 6(3), 167–191.

Geschiere, Peter (2003). Witchcraft as the dark side of kinship: Dilemmas of social security in new contexts. *Kinship*, 16(1), 43–61.

Ghosh, Debajyoti, Bernstein, Jonathan A. and Mersha, Tesfaye B. (2020). COVID-19 pandemic: The African paradox. *Journal of Global Health*, 10(2), 020348.

Goffman, E. (1963/1990). *Stigma: Notes on the Management of Spoiled Identity.* New Jersey: Prentice-Hall.

Gold Coast Government (1953). *Gold Coast Nutrition and Cookery.* London: Thomas Nelson & Sons.

Goody, Jack (ed.) (1975). *Changing Social Structure in Ghana: Essays in the Comparative Sociology of a New State and an Old Tradition.* London: International African Institute.

(1987). *The Interface between the Written and the Oral.* Cambridge: Cambridge University Press.

Gotfried, Edward A. (2014). Knowledge transmission by story telling: Malaria education of school-aged children in the Kwahu-Eastern Region, Ghana "Anansi tricks Mrs. Mosquito". *European Scientific Journal*, 10(10), 1–7.

Graboyes, Melissa (2015). *The Experiment Must Continue: Medical Research and Ethics in East Africa, 1940–2014.* Athens, OH: Ohio University Press.

Greenhalgh, Trisha and de-Graft Aikins, Ama (2023). Qualitative inquiry and public health science: Case studies from the COVID-19 pandemic. In N. K. Denzin, Y. S. Lincoln, M. D. Giardina and G. S. Cannella (eds.), *The SAGE Handbook of Qualitative Research* (6th ed.). Thousand Oaks, CA: Sage (pp. 501–518).

Grietens, Koen Peeters, Ribera, Joan M., Erhart, Annette, et al. (2014). Doctors and vampires in Sub-Saharan Africa: Ethical challenges in clinical trial research. *American Journal of Tropical Medicine and Hygiene*, 91(2), 213–215.

Guareschi, Pedrinho A. and Jovchelovitch, Sandra (2004). Participation, health and the development of community resources in southern Brazil. *Journal of Health Psychology*, 9(2), 311–322.

Guedj, Pauline (2015). The transnationalization of the Akan Religion: Religion and identity among the U.S. African American Community. *Religions*, 6(1), 24–39.

Haleegoah, J. A. S., Ruivenkamp, G., Essegbey, G., Frempong, G. and Jongerden, J. (2016). Street-vended local foods transformation: Case of Hausa Koko, Waakye and Ga Kenkey in Urban Ghana. *Advances in Applied Sociology*, 6(3), 90–100.

Helman, Cecil G. (2000). *Culture, Health and Illness.* Oxford: Butterworth-Heineman.

Hutchinson, Paul, Leyton, Alejandra, Meekers, Dominique, et al. (2020). Evaluation of a multimedia youth anti-smoking and girls' empowerment campaign: SKY girls Ghana. *BMC Public Health*, 20(1), 1–18.

International Monetary Fund (IMF) (2020). IMF Executive Board approves a US$1 billion disbursement to Ghana to address the COVID-19 Pandemic. In *IMF Country Staff Reports*, 2020 (110), 38.

Jackson, Gita (2020). A Morbid Internet Fully Embraces the Ghanaian Funeral Meme. www.vice.com (last accessed 13th April 2025).

Janzen, John M. (1978). *The Quest for Therapy: Medical Pluralism in Lower Zaire.* Berkeley: University of California Press.

Jegede, Ayodele Samuel (2007). What led to the Nigerian boycott of the polio vaccination campaign? *PLoS Medicine*, 4(3), e73.

Job, R. F. Soames (1988). Effective and ineffective use of fear in health promotion campaigns. *American Journal of Public Health*, 78(2), 163–167.

Johnson, Kim (2011). *From Tin Pan to TASPO: Steelband in Trinidad, 1939–1951*. Kingston: University Press of the West Indies.

Jovchelovitch, S. (2001). Social representations, public life and social construction. In Kay Deaux and Gina Philogene (eds.), *Representations of the Social: Bridging Theoretical Traditions*. Oxford: Blackwell (pp. 165–182).

Jovchelovitch, S. (2015). The creativity of the social: Imagination, development and social change in Rio de Janeiro's favelas. In Vlad Petre Glăveanu, Alex Gillespie and Jaan Valsiner (eds.), *Rethinking Creativity Contributions from Social and Cultural Psychology*. Hove: Routledge (pp 76–92).

Kalampalikis, Nikos and Haas, Valerie (2008). More than a theory: A new map of social thought. *Journal for the Theory of Social Behaviour*, 38(4), 449–459.

Kale, Sirin (2021). Comedian Munya Chawawa: "People think I blew up in lockdown, but I've been doing this for years". *The Guardian*, 28th November 2021.

Kalipeni, Ezekiel, Craddock, Susan, Oppong, Joseph R. and Ghosh, Jayati (eds.) (2004). *HIV and AIDS in Africa: Beyond Epidemiology*. Oxford: Blackwell Publishing.

Katz, Alfred H. (1981). Self-help and mutual aid: An emerging social movement? *Annual Review of Sociology*, 7, 129–155.

Kessler, David (2009). *The End of Overeating: Taking Control of the Insatiable American Appetite*. Emmaus: Rodale Books.

Kinney, Sylvia (1970). Drummers in Dagbon: The role of the drummer in the damba festival. *Ethnomusicology*, 14(2), 258–265.

Kok, Gergo, Peters, Gjalt-Jorn Y., Kessels, Loes T. E., et al. (2018). Ignoring theory and misinterpreting evidence: The false belief in fear appeals. *Health Psychology Review*, 12(2), 111–125.

Krause, Mariane (2003). The transformation of social representations of chronic disease in a self-help group. *Journal of Health Psychology*, 8(5), 599–615.

Kreps, Gary L. and Maibach, Edward W. (2008). Transdisciplinary science: The nexus between communication and public health. *Journal of Communication*, 58(4), 732–748.

Kroeger, Axel (1983). Anthropological and socio-medical health care research in developing countries. *Social Science and Medicine*, 17(3), 147–161.

Kummervold, Per Egil, Schulz, William S., Smout, Elizabeth, et al. (2017). Controversial Ebola vaccine trials in Ghana: A thematic analysis of critiques and rebuttals in digital news. *BMC Public Health*, 17(1), 642.

Labi, Kwame Amoah (2019). The Posuban is our Pride: Maintaining and modernising a tradition and its visual language. *Ghana Studies*, 22, 59–94.

Last, Murray (1981). The importance of knowing about not knowing. *Social Science and Medicine*, 15(3), 387–392.

Leyten, Harrie (2015). *From Idol to Art: African 'Objects with Power': A Challenge for Missionaries, Anthropologists and Museum Curators*. Leiden: African Studies Centre.

Li, Shirley (2020). Sarah Cooper has mastered the Trump joke. *The Atlantic*, 8th May 2020.

Lipinki, Jed (2013). A visit from the devil. *New York Times*. www.nytimes.com/2013/07/21/nyregion/feared-traditional-priest-from-ghana-spends-a-year-in-the-bronx-html (last accessed 13th April 2025).

Lowes, Sara and Montero, Eduardo (2021). The legacy of colonial medicine in Central Africa. *American Economic Review*, 111(4), 1284–1314.

MacPhail, Catherine and Campbell, Catherine (2001). 'I think condoms are good but, aai, I hate those things': Condom use among adolescents and young people in a Southern African township. *Social Science & Medicine*, 52(11), 1613–1627.

Maibach, Edward W., Abroms, Lorien C. and Marosits, Mark (2007). Communication and marketing as tools to cultivate the public's health: A proposed "people and places" framework. *BMC Public Health*, 7, 88.

Marfo, Kwame Asiedu (2007). Lunatics in the Takoradi central business area. *Daily Graphic*, 15th March 2007.

Markowitz, Fran and Avieli, Nir (2022). Food for the body and soul: Veganism, righteous male bodies, and culinary redemption in the Kingdom of Yah. *Ethnography*, 23(2), 181–203.

Marks, David F. (1996). Health psychology in context. *Journal of Health Psychology*, 1(1), 7–21.

Marshall, Iain J., Wolfe, Charles D. A. and McKevitt, Christopher (2012). Lay perspectives on hypertension and drug adherence: Systematic review of qualitative research. *BMJ (Online)*, 344, e3953.

Matemba, Yonah (2020). Gazing back and moving forward. *British Journal of Religious Education*, 42(2), 115–119.

McCann, James C. (2010). *Stirring the Pot: A History of African Cuisine*. Athens, OH: Ohio University Press.

McCaskie, Tom C. (2009). African American psychologists, the Atlantic slave trade and Ghana: A history of the present. In B. Rossi (ed.), *Reconfiguring Slavery: West African Trajectories*. Liverpool: Liverpool University Press (pp. 45–62).

Mensah, Joseph (2006). Cultural dimensions of globalization in Africa: A dialectical interpenetration of the local and the global. *Studies in Political Economy*, 77(1), 59–83.

Meyer, Birgit (2015). *Sensational Movies: Video, Vision and Christianity in Ghana*. Berkeley, CA: University of California Press.

Miller, Michael T. (2021). Ben Ammi's Adaptation of Veganism in the Theology of the African Hebrew Israelites of Jerusalem. *Interdisciplinary Journal for Religion and Transformation in Contemporary Society*, 9(2), 417–444.

Ministry of Health (MOH) (2012). *Regenerative Health & Nutrition: Training Manual.* Accra: MOH.

Mogaka, Ong'era F., Stewart, Jenell and Bukusi, Elizabeth (2021). Why and for whom are we decolonising global health? *Lancet*, 9(10), e1359.

Mohr, Adam (2009). Missionary medicine and Akan therapeutics: Illness, health and healing in Southern Ghana's Basel Mission, 1828–1918. *Journal of Religion in Africa*, 39(Fasc. 4), 429–461.

Moscovici, Serge (1984). The phenomenon of social representations. In R. M. Farr and S. Moscovici (eds.), *Social Representations.* Cambridge: Cambridge University Press (pp. 3–69).

(2008). *Psychoanalysis: Its Image and Its Public.* Cambridge: Polity Press.

Moscovici, Serge and Duveen, Gerard (2001). *Social Representations: Explorations in Social Psychology.* New York: New York University Press.

Mullings, Leith (1984). *Therapy, Ideology and Social Change: Mental Healing in Urban Ghana.* Berkeley, CA: University of California Press.

Nguyen, Ving-Kim (2010). *The Republic of Therapy: Triage and Sovereignty in West Africa's Time of AIDS.* Durham: Duke University Press.

Nixon, Rob (2011). *Slow Violence and the Environmentalism of the Poor.* London: Harvard University Press.

Nketia, Kwabena (1958). Akan Poetry. *Black Orpheus*, No 3, pp. 5–27.

Northern Presbyterian Agricultural Services and Partners (NPAS) (2012). Ghana's Pesticide Crisis: The Need for Further Government Action. Report, April 2012. https://reliefweb.int/report/ghana/ghana's-pesticide-crisis (last accessed 14th April 2025).

Nyantakyi-Frimpong, Hanson, Christian, Aaron K., Ganle, John and Aryeetey, Richmond (2021). "Now we've all turned to eating processed foods": A photovoice study of the food and nutrition security implications of 'galamsey' in Ghana. *Research Square*, 1–22.

Odotei, Irene (2016). Remarks on Exploring Africa's Musical Legacy. Plenary address by Emeritus Professor J. H. Kwabena Nketia. In J. H. Kwabena Nketia (ed.), *Reinstating Traditional Music in Contemporary Contexts.* Akropong-Akuapem: Regnum Africa Publications (pp. 164–165).

Oduro-Frimpong, Joseph (2014). Better Ghana agenda: On Akosua cartoons and critical public debates in contemporary Ghana. In S. Newell and O. Okome (eds.), *Popular Culture in Africa: The Episteme of Everyday.* New York: Routledge (pp. 131–154).

Ofori-Atta, Angela, Attafuah, J., Jack, H., et al. (2018). Joining psychiatric care and faith healing in a prayer camp in Ghana: Randomised trial. *British Journal of Psychiatry*, 212(1), 34–41.

Omari, Rose, Jongerden, Joost, Essegbey, George Owusu, et al. (2013). Fast food in the Greater Accra Region of Ghana: Characteristics, availability and the cuisine concept. *Food Studies: An Interdisciplinary Journal*, 1(4), 29–44.

Ortenzi, Flamina, Marten, Robert, Valentine, Nicole B., et al. (2022). Whole of government and whole of society approaches: Call for further research to improve population health and health equity. *BMJ Global Health*, 7(7), e009972.

Osseo-Asare, Abena Dove (2022). Making masks: The women behind Ghana's nose covering mandate during the COVID-19 outbreak. *Journal of Material Culture*, 28(3), 426–450.

Osseo-Asare, Fran and Baeta, Barbara (2015). *The Ghana Cookbook*. New York: Hippocrene Books.

Overholser, J. C. (2011). Collaborative empiricism, guided discovery, and the Socratic method: Core processes for effective cognitive therapy. *Clinical Psychology: Science and Practice*, 18(1), 62–66.

Pallai, EmmaLee and Tran, Kim (2019). Narrative health: Using story to explore definitions of health and address bias in health care. *The Permanente Journal*, 23, 18-052.

Panford, Solomon, Nyaney, Maud O., Amoah, Samuel O., et al. (2001). Using folk media in HIV/AIDS prevention in rural Ghana. *American Journal of Public Health*, 91(10), 1559–1562.

Park, M. P. and Park, R. H. R. (2010). Fear and humour in the art of cholera. *Journal of the Royal Society of Medicine*, 103(12), 481–483.

Parker, John (2000). The cultural politics of death and burial in early Colonial Ghana. In David M. Anderson and Richard Rathbone (eds.), *Africa's Urban Past*. Oxford: James Currey (pp. 205–221).

Patton, Sharon F. (1998). *African-American Art*. Oxford: Oxford University Press.

Pence, Alan, Makokoro, Patrick, Ebrahim, Hasina Banu and Barry, Oumar (2023). *Sankofa: Appreciating the Past in Planning the Future of Early Childhood Education, Care and Development in Africa*. Paris: UNESCO.

Perani, Judith and Smith, Fred T. (1998). *The Visual Arts of Africa: Gender, Power and Life Cycle in Africa*. Upper Saddle River, NJ: Prentice-Hall.

Philips, Keir E. J., Katagira, Winceslaus and Jones, Rupert (2020). Dance for respiratory patients in low-resource settings. *The Journal of the American Medical Association*, 324(10), 921–922.

Phillips, J. F., Awoonor-Williams, J. K., Bawah, A. A., et al. (2018). What do you do with success? The science of scaling up a health systems strengthening intervention in Ghana. *BMC Health Services Research*, 18(1), 484.

Polakoff, Claire (1978). Crafts and the concept of art in Africa. *African Arts*, 12(1), 22–23 +106.

Popkin, Barry M., Corvalan, Camila and Grummer-Strawn, Laurence M. (2019). Dynamics of the double burden of malnutrition and the changing nutrition reality. *Lancet*, 395(10217), 65–74.

Pradeilles, Rebecca, Irache, Ana, Wanjohi, Milkah N., et al. (2021). Urban physical food environments drive dietary behaviours in Ghana and Kenya: A photovoice study. *Health & Place*, 71, 102647.

PR Newswire (2022). Zlodei Agency (BADS) and Eugene Lapitsky sold the Coffin Dance meme at the NFT auction to support Ukraine. www.prnewswire.co.uk (last accessed 8th September 2023).

Quaison-Sackey, Awo A. (2021). *The Makings of a Diplomatist: The Memoirs of Alexander Quaison-Sackey*. Tema: Digibooks Ghana Ltd.
Quan-Baffour, Kofi Poku (2007). The power of Akan folk music in teaching adults about HIV/AIDS in Ghana. *Muziki*, 4(2), 209–223.
Quayson, Ato (2014). *Oxford Street, Accra: City Life and the Itineraries of Transnationalism*. Durham: Duke University Press.
Rattray, Robert S. (1955). *Ashanti*. London: Oxford University Press.
Read, Ursula M., Adiibokah, Edward and Nyame, Solomon (2009). Local suffering and the global discourse of mental health and human rights: An ethnographic study of responses to mental illness in rural Ghana. *Globalization and Health*, 5(13), 1–16.
Read, Ursula M. and Doku, Victor (2012). Mental health research in Ghana: A literature review. *Ghana Medical Journal*, 46(2), 29–38.
Rekdal, Ole Bjørn (1999). Cross-cultural healing in east African ethnography. *Medical Anthropology Quarterly*, 13(4), 458–482.
Renne, Elisha P. (2007). Mass producing food traditions for West Africans abroad. *American Anthropologist*, 109(4), 616–625.
Richards, Graham (1997). *'Race', Racism and Psychology: Towards a Reflexive History*. London: Routledge.
Robertson, Claire C. (1984). *Sharing the Same Bowl: A Socioeconomic History of Women and Class in Accra, Ghana*. Indiana University Press.
Rose, Diana (1998). Television, madness and community care. *Journal of Community and Social Psychology*, 8, 213–228.
Sarpong, Peter Kwasi (1967). The sacred stools of the Ashanti. *Anthropos*, 26(1–2), 1–60.
Scanlan, Justin Newton and Novak, Theresa (2015). Sensory approaches in mental health: A scoping review. *Australian Occupational Therapy Journal*, 62(5), 277–285.
Scharfenberger, Angela (2011). Young and wise in Accra, Ghana: A musical response to AIDS. In G. Barz and J. M. Cohen (eds.), *The Culture of AIDS in Africa: Hope and Healing through Music and the Arts*. Oxford: Oxford University Press (pp. 299–308).
Scott, Beth E., Schmidt, W. P., Aunger, R., Garbrah-Aidoo, N. and Animashaun, R. (2008). Marketing hygiene behaviours: The impact of different communication channels on reported handwashing behaviour of women in Ghana. *Health Education Research*, 24(3), 392–401.
Scott, David (1965). *Epidemic Disease in Ghana: 1901–1960*. London: Oxford University Press.
Shaban, Abdur R. A. (2020). Africa will not be vaccine testing ground: WHO slams racist French medics. *Africa News*, www.africanews.com (last accessed 8th September 2023).
Shipley, Jesse Weaver (2009). Comedians, pastors, and the miraculous agency of charisma in Ghana. *Cultural Anthropology*, 24(3), 523–552.
Singh, Arti, Owusu-Dabo, Ellis, Britton, John, Munafò, Marcus R. and Jones, Laura (2014). "Pictures don't lie, seeing is believing": Exploring attitudes to

the introduction of pictorial warnings on cigarette packs in Ghana. *Nicotine & Tobacco Research*, 16(12), 1613–1619.

Sitto, Karabo and Lubinga, Elizabeth (2020). A disease of privilege? Social representations in online media about Covid-19 among South Africans during Lockdown. *Papers on Social Representations*, 29(2), 6.1–6.29.

Sloley, Patti (2021). *Jollof Wars: Who Does West Africa's Iconic Rice Dish Best?* www.bbc.com (last accessed 15th March 2024).

Smith, Victoria Ellen (2018). *Voices of Ghana: Literary Contributions to the Ghana Broadcasting System, 1955–57* (2nd ed.). Accra: Sub-Saharan Publishers.

Sonke, Jill and Pesata, Virginia (2015). The arts and health messaging: Exploring the evidence and lessons from the 2014 Ebola outbreak. *BMJ Outcomes*, 1(1), 36–41.

Spivak, Gayatri (1988). Can the subaltern speak? In Rosalind Morris (ed.), *Can the Subaltern Speak? Reflections on the History of an Idea.* New York: Columbia University Press (pp. 21–78).

Stuckler, David and Nestle, Marion (2012). Big food, food systems, and global health. *PLoS Medicine*, 9(6), e1001242.

Stuttaford, Maria, Bryanston, Claudette, Hundt, Gillian Lewando, et al. (2006). Use of applied theatre in health research dissemination and data validation: A pilot study from South Africa. *Health: An Interdisciplinary Journal for the Social Study of Health, Illness and Medicine*, 10(1), 31–45.

Sullivan, H. (2020). 'Why should you cry?' Ghana's dancing pallbearers find new fame during COVID-19. *The Guardian*, 14th May 2020. www.theguardian.com/world/2020/may/14/why-should-you-cry-ghana's-dancing-pallbearers-find-new-fame-during-covid-19 (last accessed 14thApril 2025).

Sutherland-Addy, Esi (1998). Women and verbal arts in the Oguaa-Edina area. *Research Review (NS)*, 14(2), 1–39.

Tétrault-Farber, Gabrielle and Leo, Leroy (2023). WHO classifies EG.5 as COVID-19 "variant of interest". *Reuters*, www.reuters.com (last accessed 30th August 2023).

Tschumi, Regula and Foster, Michael (2013). The Figurative Palanquins of the Ga: History and significance. *African Arts*, 46(4), 60–73.

Tuomainen, Helena Margaret (2009). Ethnic identity, (post)colonialism and foodways: Ghanaians in London. *Food, Culture & Society*, 15(4), 526–554.

Twumasi, Patrick A. (1975). *Traditional Medical Systems in Ghana: A Study in Medical Sociology*. Tema: Ghana Publishing Corporation.

Tyler, Imogen and Slater, Tom (2018). Rethinking the sociology of stigma. *The Sociological Review Monographs*, 66(4), 721–743.

United Nations Economic Commission for Africa (UN ECA) (2020). *COVID-19 in Africa: Protecting Lives and Economies*. Addis Ababa: UN ECA.

van Andel, Tinde, Myren, Britt and van Onselen, Sabine (2012). Ghana's herbal market. *Journal of Ethnopharmacology*, 140(2), 368–378.

van der Geest, S. (2004). Dying peacefully: Considering good death and bad death in Kwahu-Tafo, Ghana. *Social Science & Medicine*, 58(5), 899–911.

Vanderpuye, Kwardua and Amegatcher, Janet (2004). Participatory HIV intervention with Ghanaian youth. In A. Singhal and W. S. Howard (eds.), *The Children of Africa Confront AIDS: From Vulnerability to Possibility*. Athens, OH: Ohio University Press (pp. 149–158).

Vokwana, Thembela (2021). *Sinikithemba* Gospel Group and the grassroots struggle against HIV/AIDS stigma in South Africa. In Bankole Falade and Mercy Murire (eds.), *Health Communication and Disease in Africa: Beliefs, Traditions and Stigma*. Singapore: Palgrave Macmillan (pp. 121–156).

Walker, Roslyn A. (2022). Five fragments of African textile history. In Christine Checinska (ed.), *Africa Fashion*. London: V&A Publishing (pp. 50–63).

Wenger, Etienne (1998). *Communities of Practice: Learning, Meaning, and Identity*. Cambridge: Cambridge University Press.

Williams-Forson, Psyche (2014). "I haven't eaten if I don't have my soup and fufu": Cultural preservation through food and foodways among Ghanaian Migrants in the United States. *Africa Today*, 61(1), 69–87.

Woets, Rhoda (2014). "This is what makes Sirigu unique" authenticating canvas and wall paintings in (inter)national circuits of value and meaning. *African Arts*, 47(4), 10–25.

Yankah, Kwesi (2004). Narrative in times of crisis: AIDS stories in Ghana. *Journal of Folklore Research*, 41(2), 181–189.

Zarocostas, John (2020). How to fight an infodemic. *Lancet*, 395(10225), 676.

Index

Accra, *17–19, 22, 26, 29–30, 38–40, 42, 48–49, 58, 67, 71, 83, 92–94, 96–97, 102, 112, 116, 118, 120–121, 131, 133, 135–136, 139–140, 146, 155, 165–166, 173, 182*
actors, *43, 59, 68, 70–71, 116*
Adzewa, *1–2, 16*
Afrobeat, *70, 92, See* music
Ahanta, *137, 176*
Akan, *3–7, 17, 21–22, 24, 30, 45, 47, 56–57, 70, 85, 110, 176*
Akufo Addo, Nana Addo Dankwa, *133*
Akwapim, also Akuapem, *6, 25, 37*
alcohol, *3–4, 22, 30, 32, 108*
Ambolley, Gyedu-Blay, *83, 171*
Ampadu, Nana Kwame, *68*
Anansesem, Ananse (Spider) stories, *70, 154, 164, See* stories
anxiety, *29, 149–150*
applied theatre, *67, 70, See* concert party, theatre
art exhibitions, *20, 96–98, 111, 153, 165*
Artists Alliance Gallery, *137, 166*
Asante, *3–4, 7, 10, 17, 49–50, 52, 57, 70, 78, 85, 87, 131, 144, 160, 181*
Ayensu, Dinah, *85*

Bambolse, *1*
beads, *3, 33–34, 162*
billboards, *40, 50, 53, 60, 62, 64, 93, 143, 156, 164*
body art, *1, 3, 46, 114*
British Museum, *5*
Brown, Horace, *58*
Brown, James, *143*

cancers, *78, 118*
  breast, *119, 125*
  liver, *78*
Cape Coast, *1*
cartoons, *20, 136, 146, 152, 156, 165*
celebrity campaign, *19, 81, 83, 164, See* mass media campaigns
check-check, *94*
cholera, *72, 150, 153, 155, 158, 160, 165*
choral music, *66, 164*
  choirs, *67, 154*
  choral groups, *66*
chronic kidney disease, *78*
chronic respiratory disease, *118, 154*
churches, *26, 31, 40, 104, 113, 133*
  Pentecostal, *26, 37, 104, 186, See* prayer camps
cognitive polyphasia, *27–28, 46*
colonial medicine, *6–7, 18, 49–50, 56*
comedians, *46, 156*
comedy, *13, 40, 44, 70–71, 131, 133, 136, 151–152, 156, 165*
  satire, *1, 44, 133, 154, 156–157*
  sketches, *20, 44, 46, 136, 156*
concert party, *70–71, 156, See* applied theatre
conscientisation, *11, 124–125*
cookery shows, *92*
copy writers, *46*
COVID arts, *20–21, 135–137, 140, 144, 151, 156–157, 159, 165, See* comedy sketches, cartoons, funeral arts, murals, songs, textiles
craft, *10, 106*
cuisines, *49–50, 83–84, 90, 92, 94–95, 162, See* recipes

Dagaba, *30*
Dagbani, *118*
Dagomba, *3–4, 17*
dance, *1–3, 6, 10, 13, 15, 40, 57, 70, 110, 114, 139, 142–143, 154, 158, 162, 170*
dance drama, *154–155, 158, 160, 165, See* applied theatre, concert party
dancing, *1, 5, 7, 66, 69, 113, 136, 138, 143, 156*
dementia, *125–126*
depression, *29, 106*
diabetes, *22–23, 26, 40–41, 44, 77–78, 118, 143, 183*
dialogical communication, *56, 159–161*
double consciousness, *149*

drums, *3–4*, *6–8*, *17*, *170*
drummers, *3*
drumming, *1*, *3*, *5*, *7*, *66*
Du Bois, W.E.B., *149*

Ebola, *57*, *59*, *146*, *150*, *152*, *180*
edutainment, *59*, *137*, *157*
Edziban Food Show, *77*, *92*, *See* cookery shows
Elmina, *1*
emotions, *12*, *17*, *25–26*, *45*, *64*, *74*, *99–100*, *106*, *114*, *117*, *152*, *162*
Ewe, *3–4*, *6*, *17*, *30*, *45*, *61*, *114*, *118*, *137*, *142*, *170–171*, *176*, *178*

Facebook, *128*, *136*
Fanon, Franz, *50*
Fante, *1–3*, *10*, *16*, *61*, *70–71*, *77*, *85*, *118*, *137*, *139*, *171–172*, *174–176*, *178*
Fantenglish, *184*
fashion, *136*, *141*, *144*, *162*
designers, 142, *162*
festivals, *2*, *7*, *15*, *17*, *30*, *32*, *35*, *46*, *100*, *162*
Aboakyer, **9**
Homowo, *4*, *32*, *85*
Odwira, *7*
film, *18*, *44*, *47–48*, *59*, *113*, *116*, *153*
folk media, *18*, *60*, *66*, *68*, *76*
Freire, Paulo, *55–56*, *125*
funerary arts, *136*, *154*, *156*
coffin design, *142*
dancing pallbearers, *136*
dirges, *66*, *136*, *142*

Ga, *4*, *7*, *10*, *17*, *24*, *29–30*, *32–33*, *37*, *40*, *45*, *61*, *85*, *94–95*, *97*, *104*, *114–115*, *118*, *137*, *142*, *171*, *174*, *176*, *178*, *181–182*
galamsey, *161*
Ghana All Stars, *60*, *171*
Gospel, *44*, *61*, *66*, *136*, *See* music
Greer, Bonnie, *5*
guinea worm, *69*

Hausa, *8*, *61*, *171*
Hayes, Isaac, *80*
heart disease, *77*, *118*, *126*
herbal clinics, *42–43*, *136*, *157*
hereditary motor sensory neuropathy, *119–120*
highlife, *61*, *66*, *83*, *104*, *136–137*, *See* music
Hip Hop, *59*, *181*, *See* music
hiplife, *61*, *66*, *136*, *149*, *151*, *181*, *See* music
HIV/AIDS campaigns, *18*, *75*, *157*
Ho, *81*, *165*
hospitals, *19*, *23–25*, *31*, *38*, *69*, *72*, *82*, *96–97*, *106*, *110–112*, *120*
hypertension, *28*, *44*, *78*, *119*, *143*

imaginaries, *45–46*, *66*, *75*, *152*, *157*
social, *66*, *152*, *157*
spiritual, *46*, *162*
Indomie, *91*, *93*
Instagram, *128*, *135*, *184*

Jamaican Patois, *61*, *171*

KFC, *90*, *92*, *94*
Kintampo, *22–23*, *39*, *97*, *104*, *113*
Klama, *32*
Koforidua, *68–69*, *73*, *157*, *164*
Konko, *68*, *73*, *75*, *154*, *157*, *164*
Kumasi, *49*, *52*, *67*, *85*, *96–97*, *118*, *131*, *136*, *141*, *164*, *181*
kwashiorkor, *40*, *69*, *182*, *See* malnutrition

LoDagaa, also Dagara, *8*, *15*, *84*

malaria, *6*, *18*, *24*, *41*, *55*, *69*, *135*, *154–155*, *158*, *160*, *164–165*
malnutrition, *78*, *80*, *94*, *159*
kwashiorkor, *40*
overnutrition, *78*
undernutrition, *78*
mass media campaigns, *53*, *60*, *63*, *67–68*, *71*, *74–76*, *156*, *See* celebrity campaigns, multi-media campaigns
McBrown's Kitchen, *92*, *See* cookery shows
mental health, *19*, *28*, *96–99*, *101–102*, *104*, *109–114*, *116*, *122*, *128–130*, *156*, *165*
mental illness, *2*, *20*, *26*, *97–101*, *104*, *106*, *111–112*, *114*, *126*, *128*, *153–154*, *156*
mixed media, *109*
mosques, *31*, *40*
Mullings, Leith, *24*, *28–31*, *37*, *45–46*, *114*, *161*
multi-media campaigns, *156*, *164–165*, *See* celebrity campaigns, mass media campaigns
multiple sclerosis, *119*
muralists, *1*, *3*, *140*
murals, *2–4*, *21*, *33*, *46*, *136*, *139–140*, *151*, *159*, *165*, *170*
music, *8*, *10*, *14*, *46*, *59*, *61*, *66*, *69–71*, *76*, *85*, *110*, *122*, *138*, *155*, *157*, *165*
musicians, *46*, *60*, *66*, *156*, *162*

Nestle, *81*, *90*
newspapers, *73–74*, *111*, *135*
adverts, *40*
cartoons, *51*
Nkoranza, *17*, *22–27*, *40*, *43*, *73*, *113*
Nubuke Foundation, *19*, *96–97*, *110*

Occupational Therapy, *96*, *See* therapies
Odotei, Irene, *4*, *10*, *32*, *36*

painting, *1, 4, 96, 100, 109, 136*
paintings, *19, 99, 106, 109, 111, 156*, *See* visual arts
photographs, *19, 101–102, 104, 111, 136, 156*
photovoice, *95, 153*
Pidgin English, *133, 137, 146, 171, 179*
Pizza Hut, *90*
poems, *55, 176*
pots, *4, 34, 86, 170*
prayer camps, *19, 26–27, 102, 104, 113, 120*, *See* churches, Pentecostal
proverbs, *2, 4, 17, 22, 66, 114, 162*
psychosis, *29*
puppetry, *66, 164*

Quashigah, Courage, *77–78*
Quashigah, Ivan, *58, 76*

R&B, *58*, *See* music
radio, *40, 46, 53, 62, 64, 67–68, 73, 76, 79, 83, 90, 93, 111, 119, 126, 144, 164*
  adverts, *40, 53*
recipes, *19, 49, 79, 81, 83–84, 87, 90, 153*, *See* cuisines
Reggae, *61, 136*, *See* music

Sankofa, *21, 161*
sculptors, *46*
sculpture, *1–2, 21, 46, 102, 142*
Seddoh Jnr, Edward, *58, 76*
seprewa, *110*
shrines, *3, 8, 16, 19, 26–27, 31, 43, 72, 104, 113–114, 157*
  Akonedi, *37*
  Posuban, *3*
  priestesses, *32, 36–37*
  priests, *32, 36, 73*
sign painters, *46*
signposts, *19, 38, 40, 46, 62, 73, 81–82, 164*
  diabetes, *39*
singing, *1, 5, 7, 40, 46, 66, 114, 138, 154, 156, 164*
Sirigu, *1*
slave trade, transatlantic, *5*
sleeping sickness, *50*
slogans, *19, 39, 46, 79, 81, 83, 90, 153, 159, 164*
smoking, *12, 65, 164–165*
songs, *4, 8, 17, 20, 45, 55, 66, 68, 75, 85, 92, 136–137, 139, 142, 152–154, 156, 176*, *See* also music
  AIDS, *66–69, 75, 154, 159*
  children's, *85, 176*
  COVID-19, *137, 142, 146, 151, 159*
  folk, *55, 142*
  ritual, *17*
  war, *8*
  women's, *1–2*
sorcery, *22, 25*
Spanish flu, *133, 135, 150*
spiritual imaginaries, *162*, *See* imaginaries
stigma, *18, 23, 60, 62–64, 71, 73–74, 87, 112, 119, 128, 144, 153, 157, 164*
  AIDS, *23, 66, 164*
  consciousness, *128, 135*
  courtesy, *23, 64, 112*
  COVID-19, *135*
stories, *1, 10, 16, 20, 43, 55, 65, 70, 72, 99, 101, 111, 115–119, 125–130, 144, 153, 156–157, 159, 162, 164*
  cancers, *118–119*
  diabetes, *116, 118*
  Ebola, *150*
  endometriosis, *119*
  hereditary motor sensory neuropathy, *119*
  hypertension, *116, 118–119*
  multiple sclerosis, *119*
  sickle-cell disease, *119*
  stroke, *116*
storytelling, *17, 20, 29, 40, 57, 66, 76, 115–118, 126, 129–130, 156*
stroke, *42, 78*
swine flu, *146, 152, 180*

Takoradi, *102*
Tallensi, also Frafra, *3*
Tamale, *78, 81, 84, 118, 155, 165*
television, *33, 40, 46, 59, 62–64, 69, 73, 76, 79, 90, 92, 120, 126, 149, 153, 155–156, 164*
  adverts, *40, 53, 90, 156*
  cookery shows, *92*
  dramas, *43, 59, 92, 153*
  programmes, *59*
  soap operas, *76, 115*
  stations, *37, 111*
textiles, *4, 133, 136, 141–142, 144, 154, 162, 165*
  designs, *1, 21, 136–137, 141, 144*
theatre, *67, 71, 75, 153*, *See* applied theatre
therapies, *14, 108*
  art therapist, *96, 114*
  art therapy, *19, 96, 98, 106, 111–112, 153*
  cognitive behavioural therapy (CBT), *108*
  diabetes self-help group, *24*
  group therapy, *108, 114*
  HIV/AIDS counselling, *62, 67*
  occupational therapist, *104*
  Occupational Therapy, *106*
  therapy damagers, *25–26*
  therapy managers, *25*
  therapy managing group, *25*
TikTok, *37*

Twi, *8*, *17*, *23*, *25*, *27*, *30*, *40*, *44*, *53*, *61*, *70*, *77*, *85*, *97*, *131*, *142*, *144*, *146*, *171*, *173–174*, *179*, *184*
Twinglish, *131*, *133*, *152*, *184*, *186*
Twitter, *44–45*, *115*, *128*, *135*, *148–149*

Unilever, *53*, *81*, *90*, *139*

visual artists, *101*
visual arts, *10*, *46*, *156*, *See* paintings

Winneba, *1*, *8*, *164*
witchcraft, *25*, *28*
woodcarvers, *4*, *10*

X, *44–45*, *94*, *115*, *135*, *149*, *186*, *See* Twitter

YouTube, *6*, *37*, *53*, *59*, *65*, *76*, *113*, *149*, *176*

Zongo, *131*, *186–187*

For EU product safety concerns, contact us at Calle de José Abascal, 56–1°, 28003 Madrid, Spain or eugpsr@cambridge.org.

www.ingramcontent.com/pod-product-compliance
Lightning Source LLC
LaVergne TN
LVHW010336220926
848484LV00004BB/908

* 9 7 8 1 0 0 9 2 4 4 4 3 5 *